CLINICAL PROBLEM SOLVING IN
PROSTHODONTICS

Commissioning Editor: Michael Parkinson
Project Development Manager: Lynn Watt
Project Manager: Nancy Arnott
Designer: Erik Bigland
Illustration Manager: Bruce Hogarth

CLINICAL PROBLEM SOLVING IN
PROSTHODONTICS

David W Bartlett BDS PhD MRD FDS RCS (restorative)

Senior Lecturer/Honorary Consultant
Department of Prosthodontics
GKT Dental Institute
London, UK

With a contribution by

Nigel F Fisher BDS FDS RCPS

Consultant/Honorary Senior Lecturer
Unit of Restorative Dentistry
GKT Dental Institute
London, UK

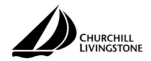

EDINBURGH LONDON NEW YORK PHILADELPHIA ST LOUIS SYDNEY TORONTO 2004

CHURCHILL LIVINGSTONE
An imprint of Elsevier Science Limited

First published 2004

ISBN 0443 072825

British Library Cataloguing in Publication Data
A catalogue record for this book is available from the British Library

Library of Congress Cataloging in Publication Data
A catalog record for this book is available from the Library of Congress

Note
Medical knowledge is constantly changing. As new information becomes available, changes in
treatment, procedures, equipment and the use of drugs become necessary. The authors and the
publishers have taken care to ensure that the information given in this text is accurate and up to
date. However, readers are strongly advised to confirm that the information, especially with regard to
drug usage, complies with the latest legislation and standards of practice.

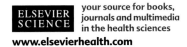

ELSEVIER SCIENCE your source for books,
journals and multimedia
in the health sciences
www.elsevierhealth.com

The
publisher's
policy is to use
**paper manufactured
from sustainable forests**

Printed in China

Preface

The learning and understanding of the concepts, as well as the subtleties, of fixed and removable prosthodontics is hugely complicated by the range and variety of problems that patients can present to their dentist. Every case is different, can be tackled in a number of ways and usually involves a variety of clinical disciplines. Added to this must be the development of dental material science, which has made a profound impact upon treatment options that have become available in many clinical situations. This book is not intended to be the definitive text on prosthodontics but the reader is encouraged to have a reasonable level of prosthodontics before using the book.

In this current environment of rapid change, the teaching of prosthodontics to senior undergraduate students, vocational and general professional trainees, as well as students undertaking specialist training, is considered by the authors to be best achieved by 'problem solving'. To this end, this book sets out a wide range of clinical situations, asks the reader to make suitable suggestions and then informs by giving considered opinions.

David W Bartlett
Nigel F Fisher

Contents

1

Vital bleaching

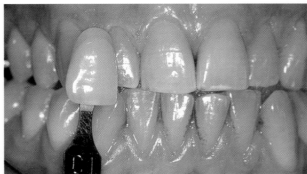

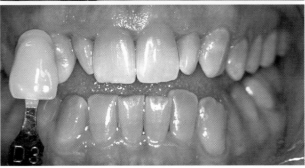

Fig. 1.2 Tetracycline stain varies in intensity from a brown–yellow discolouration to a more intense blue–grey. The more intense the staining the longer it takes to bleach the teeth; it can take up to 6 months to achieve an improvement in the appearance of the teeth. Often the cervical margin is resistant to bleaching and the overall appearance of the teeth is brighter rather than whiter.

Clinical details

A 50-year-old lady presents to your surgery complaining that her two central incisors are stained and that she would like them to match her other teeth (Fig. 1.1). She has been a smoker for 20 years and is unwilling to stop; otherwise, her medical history is clear. What treatment could you provide and what are the relative advantages and disadvantages of each method?

Clinical observations

- The periodontal condition is good.
- The stain remains despite a thorough prophylaxis.
- The patient is not concerned about the colour match of the crown on the maxillary premolar.
- The shade guide has been used to show the patient the original colour before any treatment has been commenced.
- All the maxillary and mandibular incisors are unrestored and gave a vital response to the electric pulp test.
- The cause of the staining remains unclear but may be related to the smoking.

Complicating factors

Smoking may continue to discolour the teeth and the patient needs to be informed of this possibility.

The patient has a high lip line and when smiling shows the gingival margins of the maxillary incisor teeth.

Although the diagnosis remains unclear, what are the potential causes of this discolouration?

Extrinsic staining.
Tetracycline (Fig. 1.2).
Hereditary causes (e.g. dentinogenesis imperfecta, amelogenesis imperfecta).
Fluoride (Fig. 1.3).
Loss of vitality.

Hereditary causes are unlikely as the effects would be widespread, similarly so for both fluoride and tetracycline staining. Although fluoride and tetracycline staining can be more localized, all teeth developing at the time of administration of the tetracycline or fluoride would be affected. It would be reasonable to suppose, therefore, that the first molars would be stained, but this was not the case. As the staining is localized, smoking was identified as the most likely cause.

What are the options for treatment to improve the appearance of the teeth?

Bleaching.
Veneers.
Crowns.

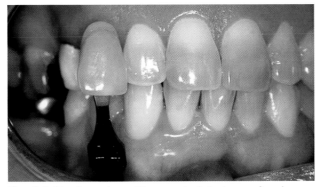

Fig. 1.1 Discoloured maxillary central incisors of unknown aetiology.

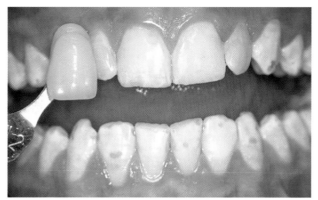

Fig. 1.3 Fluorosis usually presents as brown and white localized speckles, together with an overall whiter appearance of the enamel surface. The brown discolouration is normally whitened with bleaching but the whiter areas are often more resistant.

● Bleaching

Darkening of teeth caused by ageing is possibly one of the more common forms of discoloured teeth and may be successfully treated with vital bleaching. Although the cause of age-related stains is often difficult to identify, it is suspected that the darker colour is formed following wear of the enamel, so exposing the underlying yellow colour of dentine. Dentine itself also tends to darken with age. Vital bleaching relies upon the action of hydrogen peroxide products which are applied, for extended times, close to the tooth surfaces. The superoxide ion, which is released from the rapidly decaying hydrogen peroxide molecule, is highly reactive and breaks down stains of organic origin within the enamel and dentine (Fig. 1.4).

Successful bleaching needs good case selection (Fig. 1.5). Different people perceive colour differently and what appears acceptable to one person may not be to someone else. The most commonly researched vital bleaching products are those containing a 10% solution of carbamide peroxide. This material breaks down to form a 3% solution of hydrogen peroxide and urea. [At the time of writing, the legalization regarding the use of carbamide peroxide that delivers levels above 0.1% hydrogen peroxide is unclear.] The carbamide peroxide is usually delivered in a viscous gel that is applied closely to

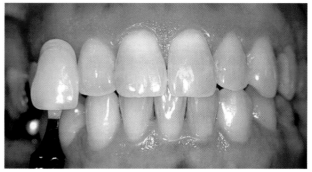

Fig. 1.4 Treatment completed. The patient had vital bleaching using carbamide peroxide placed in a vacuum-formed appliance and used the system for 3 weeks.

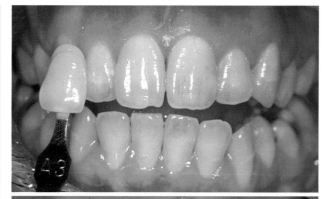

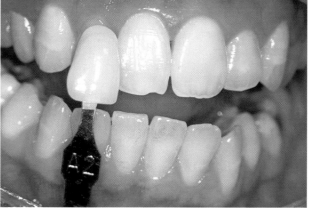

Fig. 1.5 Bleaching should be considered on teeth with small or preferably no restorations. The most successful results are usually achieved with age-related changes or when a slight change in tooth colour is requested. Intense stains take longer to whiten.

the teeth in a custom-made, vacuum-formed tray. The appliance should be contoured to just below the gingival margins to reduce the potential for gingival irritation which might result from seepage of peroxide. A spacer, commonly die relief, is applied to the study model of the teeth needing bleaching. The thickness of the tray should be around 1 mm, not so thick that it causes discomfort.

These products are most successful if the patient wears the trays, loaded with the peroxide, for up to 3–4 hours a day for about a month. This is usually in the evening and can sometimes be extended overnight. The application time may differ between products. For more intense stains, such as those from tetracycline, it may take 3–6 months to produce a successful result. If patients do not use the product each day there is insufficient time for the hydrogen peroxide to bleach the teeth. It is helpful before treatment to use a shade guide to match to the stained teeth and, if possible, to take a photograph of the teeth for the patient's records. Some manufacturers supply 'power bleaching' products, which contain a more concentrated hydrogen peroxide; these bleach teeth at the chair side. Home bleaching and 'power bleaching' can be used in conjunction to provide an acceptable clinical result. There is some advantage to power bleaching as the dentist maintains control of the bleaching product and does not have to rely on the patient's motivation and compliance with instructions.

A relatively common complication of vital bleaching is cervical dentine sensitivity. If this becomes a problem, the treatment should be discontinued. Some patients are willing to accept a minor degree of discomfort in an effort to achieve a change in colour of their teeth. Another possible complication is that the effects of the bleaching may reverse. This varies with each patient and is impossible to predict.

● Veneers

Composite or porcelain veneers cemented to the labial surfaces of the maxillary incisors will improve the appearance of the stained teeth. In this case, the high lip line may make the margin of the veneers visible when the patient smiles. Although this might not be an immediate problem, the cement margins of the veneer can take up stain and become visible (Fig. 1.6). Stain can develop either as a result of a breakdown and uptake of dietary products into the composite lute or from caries developing at or beneath the margin.

Veneer preparations can either be finished close to the incisal edge (Fig. 1.7) or the incisal edge of the tooth reduced in height by 1 mm or more to permit an overlap. The latter is usually preferred by the dental technician because it allows for the introduction of a translucent porcelain incisal edge. However, by taking the veneer over the incisal edge and onto the palatal surface there is a risk that the porcelain may fracture from high loading forces of the opposing teeth, especially during anterior excursive movements of the mandible.

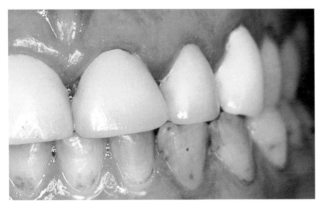

Fig. 1.6 These veneers, from another patient, have failed for a variety of reasons. The colour of the veneer is too opaque and could have been improved with more translucent cements. Some manufacturers produce water-soluble try-in pastes, allowing the dentist to estimate the appearance of the veneer after cementation. These veneers were 5 years old and had begun to stain around the margins. The mesial surface of the central incisor shows some underlying dentine, emphasizing the problem of undercuts on curved teeth. The technician has been unable to finish the porcelain around the mesial surface to overcome this and more tooth preparation is needed to reduce the curvature of the tooth and eliminate the undercuts. The gingival condition has also deteriorated partly from the deficient margins and also from the patient suffering from xerostomia.

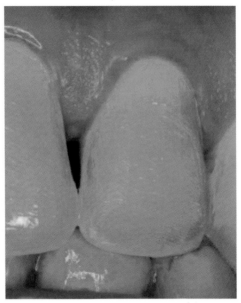

Fig. 1.7 Veneer preparation on a lateral incisor. The contact point is maintained and the finish line has not passed onto the palatal aspect along the incisal edge.

Another potential problem with indirect veneer techniques is that undercuts can be inadvertently created on the interproximal surfaces of canines and teeth with significant convex shapes, making the laboratory production difficult. Further tooth preparation would be necessary to remove the undercuts. Imbricated incisors will also introduce undercuts between adjacent teeth, making veneers contraindicated (Fig. 1.8).

Making temporary restorations for indirect veneers is difficult without compromising the prepared surface for the definitive restoration. If a dentine-bonding agent is used to retain the temporary restoration, the surface becomes contaminated and a clean bond between definitive restoration and the tooth cannot be achieved.

Ideally, preparations for indirect veneers should not pass through the contact points on adjacent teeth because, unless the veneers are cemented within a very short time,

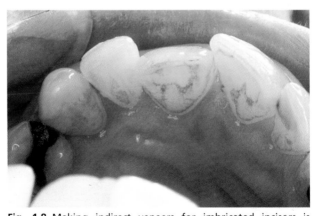

Fig. 1.8 Making indirect veneers for imbricated incisors is contraindicated without preparing the interproximal surfaces, which might then drift between the time of preparation and fit of the veneers.

drifting and closure of the gap can occur, so preventing the accurate fitting of the veneers. The appearance of indirect veneers can be excellent and generally superior to direct veneers, which can appear monochromatic. Recently, some manufacturers have overcome this problem by manufacturing micro hybrid composites with a range of shades and opacities, giving the clinician greater control over the final appearance of the restoration.

● Crowns

Conventional crowns in this case would normally be considered overly destructive. In particular, metal–ceramic crowns can often appear bright and slightly opaque. This is because the construction of this type of crown requires an inner metal coping of between 0.3 and 0.5 mm thickness covered by an opaque porcelain layer of 0.3 mm. On top of this is applied the aesthetic veneering ceramic. To accommodate these three layers in a manner that allows for a sufficient thickness for the veneering ceramic to produce a natural-looking result requires substantial tooth preparation. The risk of damage to the pulp can be significant. All-ceramic crowns can often produce an aesthetic result superior to metal–ceramic crowns and should be considered when an optimum cosmetic result is essential.

Learning outcomes

● Able to differentiate the causes of discoloured teeth.
● Management of discoloured teeth using vital bleaching techniques.
● Understand the action of hydrogen peroxide.
● Complications of using indirect anterior veneers and full coverage crowns.

2

Non-vital bleaching

Clinical details

This patient attends your clinic requesting a crown on the maxillary discoloured central incisor (Fig. 2.1). There are no medical complications. The tooth was traumatized 6 years ago and root-treated soon after, but has gradually discoloured over the succeeding years. The patient's adjacent teeth are unrestored and otherwise the dentition is unrestored. What will be your advice and give reasons for your treatment.

Clinical observations

- There is no radiographic evidence of apical pathology and the tooth is symptomless.
- The obturation of the root canal is satisfactory.
- The coronal seal is intact.
- There is no clinical evidence of periodontal disease or caries.
- The diagnosis of the staining is a non-vital tooth.

Complicating factors

There are no complicating factors.

Why do non-vital teeth stain?

The most likely cause of the discolouration is the breakdown of blood pigments within the dentine–pulpal complex. The haemoglobin breaks down to produce the stains associated with the darkening. The severity of the discolouration varies between patients, but can be very

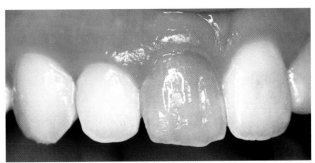

Fig. 2.1 A non-vital discoloured incisor.

intense. An additional cause can be bacterial leakage between coronal restorations and the pulp chamber. This may explain why some root-filled teeth can discolour years after root canal treatment. Even the darkest stained teeth can respond well to non-vital bleaching techniques.

What are the options for treatment in this case?

Non-vital bleaching.
Veneer.
Crown.

● Non-vital bleaching

Like vital bleaching, the active agent is hydrogen peroxide. Any tooth considered for non-vital bleaching should have an intact coronal seal, be well obturated with gutta percha and have no radiographic evidence of disease.

Gutta percha should be removed to below the level of the gingival margin in the root canals and any remaining restorative material, such as composite, removed from the buccal surface of the access cavity. It is important to use a non-end-cutting bur to safely remove the gutta percha to a level 3–4 mm down the root canal to prevent the possibility of stain remaining around the cervical margin of the tooth.

It is important to ensure that an adequate seal is present both apically and coronally. There is a potential for some leakage of the hydrogen peroxide towards the apical tissues and a hard base is likely to reduce that risk. The hard base can be made from glass ionomer, zinc phosphate or a composite, and should be placed above the gutta percha to seal the canal from the bleaching agent. A slurry of sodium perborate and 30% (100 vols) hydrogen peroxide is placed into the access chamber, which is sealed with cotton wool and a temporary cement (Fig. 2.2). An alternative is to use a proprietary bleaching agent such as 35% carbamide peroxide. The temporary material can be made from zinc oxide–eugenol, polycarbonate, glass ionomer or composite. The patient is reviewed within 2 weeks and the process repeated until the colour is improved to the patient's satisfaction (Fig. 2.3). The results are usually seen within a few weeks, but if it is not successful within that time other options should be considered. Often the most resistant site for bleaching is around the cervical margin and onto the root surface. This area remains dark and resistant even to prolonged bleaching. The other options for improving the appearance were discussed in Case 1.

● Veneer

It is difficult to match single porcelain restorations to natural teeth. Masking severely darkened non-vital teeth with either direct or indirect restorations is also problematic. Moderately darkened teeth can usually be restored with a combination of an opaque luting cement

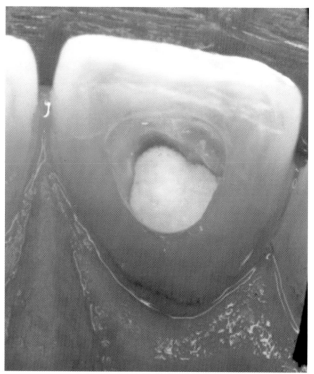

Fig. 2.2 The gutta percha must be removed from the root canal and to a depth below the gingival margin. This will ensure that the hydrogen peroxide can reach all parts of the coronal tooth tissue. Further reduction is needed apically to provide sufficient space for a base.

and a porcelain veneer that has a layer of opaque porcelain on the fit surface, but this will increase the thickness of the veneer. Too thick a veneer will produce a labial protuberance of the restoration and affect its appearance.

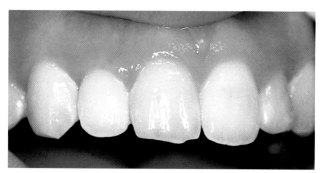

Fig. 2.3 The bleached tooth nearly matches the adjacent one and is sufficiently lighter for patient acceptance.

● Crown

Normally a metal–ceramic crown needs a 1.5-mm preparation on the buccal surface to create sufficient space for the metal and the porcelain. If 1.5 mm is removed from this buccal surface there might not be sufficient bulk of the remaining tooth to support the core, and a post would then be needed to support a crown. Bleaching the tooth improves the appearance and eliminates the need for a crown. What makes bleaching the ideal treatment for this tooth is that it is otherwise unrestored.

Learning outcomes

- To understand why non-vital teeth stain.
- How to bleach non-vital teeth.
- To appreciate the difficulties of restoring root-treated upper incisors.

3

All-ceramic crowns

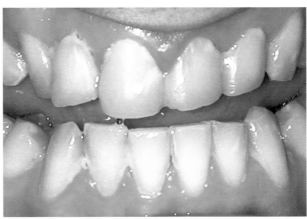

Fig. 3.1 These discoloured anterior composites are poorly shaped, stained and need replacing.

Clinical details

This 46-year-old woman is dissatisfied with the appearance of her composite veneers (Fig. 3.1). They appear to be lifeless and stained and she would like them replaced.

Clinical observations

- She has a moderately restored dentition.
- There is no active periodontal disease or caries.
- The incisal relationship is Class I.
- Periapical radiographs of the teeth show no apical changes and pulp-vitality tests give a positive response.
- The diagnosis of the staining is deterioration of the existing composite veneers by partial leakage around the margins of the restoration and wear of the material sufficient to require replacement.

What are the options for treatment?

Replace with metal–ceramic crowns.
Replace with all-porcelain crowns.
Leave alone and monitor.

All-porcelain crowns usually have a better appearance than metal–ceramic ones, but the end result will depend to a great extent upon the technician. Both types of crown will need significant amounts of tooth reduction and neither could be considered conservative of tooth tissue.

What impression technique should you use?

The most commonly used impression materials for fixed prosthodontics are polyethers or silicones (Box 3.1). Manufacturers claim that polyethers are hydrophilic, yet they still require a dry and clean preparation. Silicones are generally accepted to be slightly less hydrophilic, but recently some manufacturers have introduced more hydrophilic silicones.

The need for gingival retraction will depend upon individual circumstances. If the preparation is supragingival or at the gingival margin there is probably no need. Subgingival preparations need gingival retraction, partly to prevent bleeding but also to act as a physical barrier and retract the gingival tissues.

Box 3.1 Impression materials for crown and bridges

Silicone (addition cured)
This is probably the most commonly used impression material in general practice. It is elastic and reasonably rigid and is available in a variety of formulations: gun delivery systems with a low, medium or high viscosity or putty–wash mix. Most of the impression materials are hydrophobic and do not take good impressions in wet conditions. Silicone is a very accurate material and dimensionally stable over long periods of time. Most manufacturers use different contrasting colours for two-phase impressions but recently a few have introduced one-phase materials similar in texture and viscosity to a well-known polyether material.

Polyether
Unlike silicones, polyethers have a higher rigidity and make particularly good impressions for implants because of their resistance to tearing. The material is not stable in wet conditions and must be stored dry. It is particularly rigid and sometimes liable to tearing. Bridges or mobile teeth may be inadvertently removed or extracted if they have not been blocked-out prior to taking the impression.

Hydrocolloids
Practitioners, mainly because of the cost of the system, rarely use reversible hydrocolloids. Irreversible hydrocolloids are commonly used for the opposing impressions but lack sufficient accuracy. Irreversible hydrocolloid impressions need casting within an hour as they quickly become susceptible to moisture changes in the atmosphere.

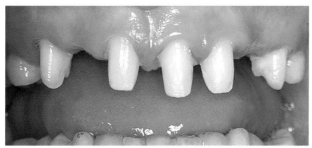

Fig. 3.2 These preparations are correctly prepared to provide sufficient retention for conventional metal-ceramic crowns. There is a sharp mesial angle on UR1 which would make the use of a Procera scanner difficult.

Special trays are generally not required so long as the chosen stock trays are sufficiently rigid. There is little difference in the accuracy of an impression when using a metal or rigid-plastic stock tray. Stock trays made from flexible plastic are not suitable as they will flex under load and distort the impression. Stock trays are usually perforated. A special tray is necessary when the arch form is grossly abnormal (e.g. repaired cleft palates or when the arch is much longer or wider than can be accommodated by a stock tray). Difficulties can often arise when trying to take an impression of a last standing molar because the impression can often 'drag' distally. Usually, a stock tray can be modified by the addition of acrylic resin or impression compound distally to cover the single standing tooth.

How do conventional crowns gain retention?

Conventional crowns gain retention from the shape of the preparation (Fig. 3.2). Adhesively cemented crowns rely on the lute to provide the retention. The length and taper of a preparation are the most important factors in the retention of conventionally cemented crowns. Most crowns are placed with a vertical path of insertion. To unseat a crown it must either be pulled off in the same direction, by the patient chewing sticky foods or by the dentist. In most cases the taper achieved should be between 10° and 15°. Short clinical crowns create problems of retention and will be discussed later. A long preparation can also create problems. Increasing the length of the preparation increases the risk of introducing undercuts, which can in turn make the crown difficult to fit.

Where do you finish the gingival margins for crowns?

The margins of crowns placed at or just below the gingival margin will have a less damaging effect on the periodontal tissues and yet maintain a satisfactory appearance compared to crown margins placed subgingivally. A subgingival margin encourages plaque build-up, hindering adequate access to tooth-brushing and increasing the potential for periodontal disease. The medium- to long-term result might be recession of the gingival tissues and exposure of the margin of the crown. It is better that the dentist places the crown margin supragingivally if the appearance is not important or just below the gingival sulcus to allow cleaning and reduce the potential for periodontal disease. If the margin must be placed subgingivally if should be placed at half the depth of a healthy gingival sulcus.

The preparation should follow the natural contour of the gingival tissues and is particularly demanding interproximally. A common finding with preparations is that the margin is cut in a single plane rather than following the gingival contour. This results in sectioning of the interdental connective tissue attachment from which follows papillary recession, causing the familiar 'punched-out' appearance between crowns. An additional complication is often buccal gingival recession which exposes crown margins previously buried beneath the gingival tissues. The other relevant feature around the margin is the emergence angle of the crown. If the crown is made too bulbous it becomes over-contoured and pushes the gingival tissues outwards. This increases the risk for plaque retention and the development of periodontal disease. Conversely, if the crown is under-contoured the appearance is compromised in an important area.

Porcelain has a weak fracture resistance in thin section and therefore the margin should be prepared to butt joint. To improve the appearance of metal crowns the metal can be cut back from the buccal surface and the margin finished in porcelain. This improves the translucency of the restoration at this most critical surface.

What types of porcelain crowns are commonly available?

High-strength cores.
Pressed-glass ceramics.
Milled porcelains.
Capillary technique.
CAD–CAM.
Metal–ceramic.

● High-strength cores

e.g. Inceram (Vita Zahnfabrik, Bad Sackingen, Germany) The crown consists of two layers. The crown's strength is derived from the inner core made from Inceram, which is a glass and alumina material, and overlaid with conventional porcelains to improve the appearance. Fine alumina powder is applied to an absorbent refractory die and any residual pores are filled with molten glass to produce a dense, crystalline core structure. The core has high strength and elastic modulus, but the improved strength is sacrificed for a poor appearance. Additionally, the high content of alumina makes it resistant to most acids, making adhesive bonding difficult; thus non-adhesive cement is used to cement the crowns (Fig. 3.3).

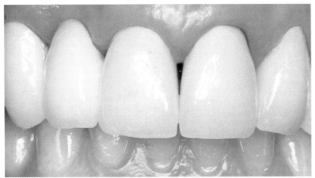

Fig. 3.3 Inceram crowns. These very hard crowns allow light to diffuse through and so remain translucent, but their monochromatic colour can make them appear a little bright.

Inceram crowns were among the first generation of the newer all-ceramic crowns and can produce acceptable results. However, unlike the newer developments, the crown retains a rather glass-like appearance, although this is balanced by its reportedly high strength.

● Pressed-glass ceramics

e.g. Empress (Ivoclar Vivadent, Schaan, Liechtenstein)
Like Inceram crowns, the crown comprises two layers: an inner material made from Empress and an outer layer made from conventional porcelains. The outer layer is thinner than in Inceram crowns; this is needed to improve the surface finish and characteristics rather than to make the crown's appearance acceptable. The Empress core is made using the lost-wax technique. Wax is applied to a phosphate-bonded investment material and, after burn-out, a leucite-reinforced glass ceramic is pressed under pressure into the space left by the wax (Fig. 3.4). The fit surface can be acid-etched with hydrofluoric acid to allow adhesive bonding.

Unlike milled ceramics such as Procera, pressed-glass ceramics are homogeneous. Most teeth have a complex colour consisting of a variety of shades. However, the bulk of an Empress crown is monochromatic and,

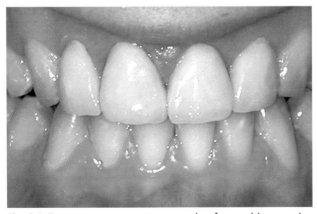

Fig. 3.4 Empress crowns are an example of pressable ceramics. The crown is made using the principles of the lost wax technique. Most of the crown is made from Empress apart from the surface finish.

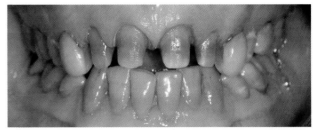

Fig. 3.5 Preparations for Procera crowns (Nobel Biocare, Sweden). Ideally, crown preparations should have rounded surfaces to allow the laser scanner to digitize the model surface accurately. Sharp angles are poorly recorded.

although some individual characteristics are possible to build into the outer layer of the crown with porcelain, the inner shade remains the same.

● Milled-porcelain cores

Procera (Nobel Biocare, Gothenburg, Sweden)
The concept is not unlike that of Inceram, but in this case computer-controlled technology is used to mill the coping to a pre-determined thickness. The working die is scanned by a sapphire probe and converted into data which is digitized and sent by e-mail to a laboratory with a computer-controlled milling machine. The ingot is made from an aluminium oxide powder. The outer surface, like Inceram crowns, is made from conventional porcelain (Figs 3.5 and 3.6).

The fit of these crowns is normally excellent because of the milling techniques used to manufacturer the core. Conventional ceramic is overlaid onto the core and is responsible for the improved translucency compared to metal–ceramic crowns. The material can be adhesively bonded to teeth. Procera porcelain can be used to make simple three-unit bridges (Fig. 3.7) or veneers.

● Capillary techniques

Captek (Schottlander & Davis, Letchworth, UK)
The crown's basic structure is similar to conventional metal–ceramic crowns except that the core is made from a precious metal. A series of wax strips, impregnated

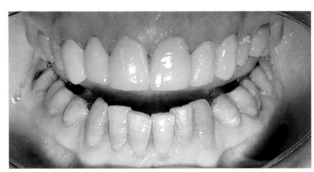

Fig. 3.6 The definitive Procera crowns fitted for the patient in Fig. 3.5. The crowns have a hard and strong inner core, but overlying it is conventional porcelain which provides the characteristics of the tooth. The marginal fit of these crowns is generally accepted to be particularly good.

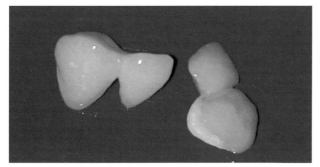

Fig. 3.7 Procera bridges. An all-ceramic simple cantilever bridge crown is made by cementing a preformed pontic onto the retainer. This often means that the interdental contact is long or broad, which might affect the appearance.

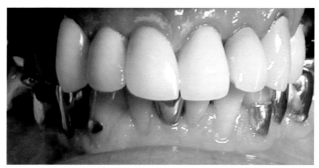

Fig. 3.8 Captek crowns are made by layering gold- and palladium-enriched waxes to create a core, over which is placed conventional porcelain. The strong core can make this type of crown conservative of tooth tissue. The crowns on UL2 and UL3 are metal–ceramic; those on UL1 to UR3 are Captek.

with gold and platinum, are applied to a refractory die. The die is heated to burn off the wax, leaving a metallic substructure over which porcelain is applied to produce the crown.

These crowns are reported to have improved marginal fit and biocompatibility. Their appearance is usually warmer than that of conventional metal-ceramic crowns because the yellow colour from the gold core reflects the light (Fig. 3.8). They are reported to require less buccal/facial reduction and are therefore more conservative of tooth tissue. Until recently, adhesively bonding precious alloys to teeth was unreliable, but a recent material has overcome this problem (Panavia F: Kuraray, Japan).

● CAD–CAM

Computer-aided design/computer-aided manufacturing systems cut blocks of porcelain to produce inlays or crowns from digitized images of crown preparations. This method uses conventional porcelains but they are manufactured uniquely. Although this technique has been available for some time, its use in general practice is fairly limited, although the technique might become more widespread in the future as technology develops.

● Metal–ceramic

The conventional and most commonly used technique utilizes the bond between porcelain and metal that is achieved at high temperatures. The type of metal can vary from high gold/low non-precious metal to low gold/high palladium or non-precious metal. The higher the palladium

alloy the harder it is to solder units together (Table 3.1). Sufficient space is needed from the tooth preparation to allow for the opaque porcelain, which bonds to the metal, and the conventional porcelain which creates the appearance.

What cement lute should you choose?

For most conventionally prepared teeth the choice of cement lute is normally arbitrary and depends on individual preferences. There is some benefit in using non-adhesive cements as they possess a degree of retrievability, but there is probably little clinical difference in using a glass ionomer cement and, say, zinc phosphate, apart from fluoride leach with the former. Adhesive cements will improve the retention of short clinical crowns. The choice of cement for luting all porcelain crowns is shown in Table 3.2.

How do you take the shade of a crown?

Shade taking can vary in complexity, from a single shade taken from a guide to the inclusion of surface characteristics and custom-made guides if individual features need to be incorporated. In most cases, the shade should be taken in natural daylight or daylight-producing lamps and at the beginning of the appointment. Quick glances at the natural tooth colour will produce the best match, as the retina rapidly becomes bleached with prolonged staring, which distorts colour perception. Ensure that there are no bright colours immediately adjacent (e.g. lipstick, clothing). The most difficult tooth to match is a

Table 3.1 Characteristics of gold alloys

Gold type	% gold	Consistency	Stress level	Examples
1	85	Soft	Low	Small inlays
2	75	Medium	Moderate	Onlays/inlays
3	70	Hard	High	Onlays, thin castings, full crowns
4	65	Extra hard	Extra high	Clasps, crowns, denture framework

Table 3.2 Which luting cement to use for cementing crowns

Adhesive cements	Non-adhesive cements (including glass ionomers)
Procera	Metal–ceramic
Empress	Inceram
Metal–ceramic	
Captek	

single crown in an otherwise unrestored dentition, especially an upper incisor.

Ideally, the technician should be involved with the shade selection, but this is not always feasible and the clinician will need to provide a suitable prescription. This is generally accomplished by using a porcelain manufacturer's shade guide. The one most commonly used is Vita Lumin Vacuum (now renamed Vitapan Classical). It is reasonably logical in layout and simple to use. Of the four sections A, B, C and D, A hues are orange, B hues are yellow, C greyish yellow and D greyish red. Each section increases chroma from 1 to 4. The majority of natural teeth will fall within this range.

A short look at several natural teeth will usually indicate the hue as mainly orange or yellow; thus the initial selection is made from A or B, with the appropriate degree of chroma. For lower value (greyer) versions of A shades, select from group D; for lower value B shades, select from group C.

It is very helpful to make a drawing of the tooth to be crowned and indicate particular characteristics to be incorporated (neck effect, incisal translucency, check lines, etc.) and to specify the surface texture and level of glaze, as these factors will have considerable influence on how natural the finished crown will appear.

Learning outcomes

● Managing failing anterior restorations.
● Understanding the principles of preparing crowns.
● Selecting all-ceramic crowns.
● Cementing crowns.
● How to take a shade.
● Choice of impression materials for making crowns and bridges.

4

Ceramic onlays

Clinical details

This patient suffers from regurgitation erosion and needs restorations on his premolars as part of a more complicated treatment plan (Fig. 4.1). There are no medical complications and his symptoms of reflux have recently been controlled with medication.

Clinical observations

- Both teeth give a positive response to the electric pulp tester.
- There is sufficient interocclusal space for the restorations.
- The restorations are part of a full mouth rehabilitation.
- The diagnosis of the tooth wear is regurgitation erosion and a parafunctional activity.

What are the options for treatment?

Direct composite build-ups.
Indirect composite, porcelain or metal onlays.
Amalgam restorations.
Glass ionomer.
Elective root treatment with conventional post and core.

● Direct composite build-ups

These are the simplest restorations and rely upon the strength of the bond between the tooth and dentine-bonding agent/composite to retain the restoration. Thereafter, the composite can be used as a core for a conventional crown or used as the definitive treatment. The advantage of using a composite and a dentine-bonding agent linked to the tooth is the high bond strength, which is sufficient for retention. Additional forms, such as pins or grooves, are not needed. In addition, because the bond is the major retentive feature, removal of tooth tissue is only required if caries is present and it is therefore a more conservative technique.

Direct composite can be difficult to place, especially around contact points. Although there are a number of recent matrix bands, which are reportedly easier to use and produce a more consistent contact point, this still remains a clinically demanding technique.

The core is retained between the dentine-bonding agent and the tooth surface. Most modern dentine-bonding agents have approximately similar bond strengths to enamel and dentine. It is believed that the strength of the bond results from the micro-mechanical tags of the bonding agent penetrating the dentinal tubules and infiltrating the hybrid layer. The hybrid layer is the partially demineralized surface of the dentine, which acts somewhat like a sponge and into which the low-viscosity resins penetrate.

● Indirect onlays

Either composite, porcelain or metal-based onlays can be used to restore the coronal surfaces. Again, these materials rely on the bond strength between the dentine-bonding agent and the tooth to retain the restoration.

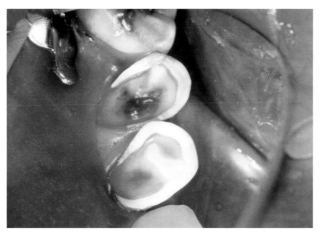

Fig. 4.1 The pre-operative appearance of the patient in Case 4. Restoring the palatal surfaces eroded by gastric acid can be achieved with direct or indirect adhesively bonded materials, a pinned amalgam, glass ionomer or an elective root treatment.

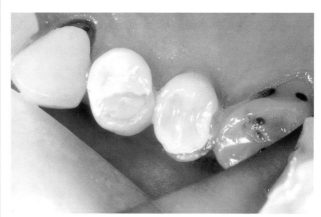

Fig. 4.2 These teeth were restored with an indirect porcelain retained to the teeth by a luting cement using a dentine-bonding agent.

The advantage of an indirect technique is that the technician controls the contact points (Fig. 4.2). Maintaining contact points with direct techniques can be difficult, especially when there is little tooth tissue remaining.

Recent developments in indirect composites have overcome the early problems of staining and fractures. Together with all ceramics, the most important principle is to ensure that onlays are sufficiently thick to resist fracture. Porcelain and indirect composites are weak in thin section. Therefore, at least 2 mm of interocclusal space should be left to overcome this problem.

● Amalgam

In the present case, the cavity lacks conventional retention, which would be needed for an amalgam. Therefore undercuts would be necessary underneath the buccal cusp and probably a pin on the palatal margin. The use of pins has reduced over recent years because of the development of adhesives; however, it is generally not prudent to rely upon the adhesive bond between amalgam and tooth to provide retention of a restoration. Pins, slots and grooves and undercuts, where appropriate, are still needed to create the necessary retention for amalgam restorations.

In this case, substantial amounts of tooth would need removing to create an undercut on the buccal wall, together with pins and grooves to aid retention of an amalgam. Therefore, it is not the most appropriate material to use to restore this tooth. If an amalgam were used it would almost certainly need a three-quarter crown for its final restoration.

● Glass ionomers

Glass ionomers adhere to enamel and dentine, but their bond strengths do not approach those of dentine-bonding agents. Some clinicians use sandwich restorations to restore broken-down teeth. The area of dentine exposure combined with the relatively low bond strength between the glass ionomer and the dentine is unlikely to be strong enough to retain the restoration. Even the benefit of the composite bonding to the enamel may not overcome this problem. But, more importantly, the glass ionomer will dissolve in the acid originating from the stomach. Therefore, glass ionomers should not be used in patients with dietary or regurgitation erosion.

● Elective root treatments

An elective root treatment would be particularly destructive and remove significant amounts of tooth tissue in a patient who has an already compromised dentition. The coronal access would necessitate removal of substantial amounts of dentine in a patient who has attrition. There would be an increased likelihood of a root fracture in a patient with a parafunctional habit.

Learning outcomes

● Assessing and restoring broken-down teeth.

5

Managing occlusal changes

Clinical details

This 48-year-old man presents to you with continually fracturing and breaking down posterior teeth and would like it to stop (Fig. 5.1). He had a number of teeth extracted about 10 years ago and has noticed that the teeth have continually fractured over the last few years. There are no medical problems and he is fit and healthy. What are the potential complications from extracting the teeth? What are your treatment options?

Clinical observations

- There is no bleeding on probing and the probing depths are within normal limits.
- He has an extensively restored dentition with a few missing teeth.
- The lower left first molar was extracted some 10 years ago; the second molar has tilted mesially and the upper first molar has over-erupted into the space left by the missing tooth.
- The patient has a canine-guided occlusion.
- The patient is a smoker.

What are the potential complications in treatment?

The mesial movement of the lower molar and the downward movement of the upper premolar and molar

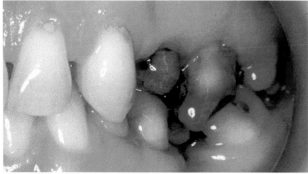

Fig. 5.1 This unstable occlusion resulted after the lower molar was extracted and the opposing and adjacent teeth drifted into the edentulous space. (Courtesy Dr David Ricketts.)

have introduced occlusal interferences. Such an unstable occlusion gives the potential for high, laterally directed forces to be applied to the posterior and anterior teeth alike. Teeth with existing large restorations are particularly prone to fracture of their cusps or restorations.

In some patients who are susceptible to mandibular dysfunction, an occlusal interference may trigger symptoms of pain, jaw-joint clicking or restriction of mandibular movement. If the symptoms become chronic, one of the first lines of treatment is to provide an occlusal splint. A well-established type of appliance is the Michigan splint. This is made from heat-cured, clear acrylic resin and is designed to cover all the occlusal and incisal surfaces of the maxillary teeth (Fig. 5.2). The splint is adjusted to provide even and interference-free contact with the mandibular dentition and should be worn over-night until the symptoms abate. If this treatment provides relief from symptoms, either the Michigan splint becomes the definitive treatment or occlusal adjustment is undertaken to eliminate the interference and, in theory, keep the patient symptom-free. If the patient does not respond to the Michigan splint (see Box 5.1), other, non-dental, causes should be investigated. The definitions of occlusal positions are shown below.

The appearance in this present case has been described as an unstable occlusion and can be considered

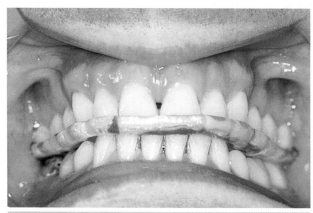

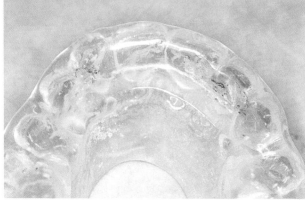

Fig. 5.2 The Michigan splint is a full-coverage, hard acrylic, maxillary splint made so that there is even posterior occlusal contact with shared anterior guidance and canine-guided lateral excursions.

Box 5.1 The Michigan splint

These full-coverage maxillary splints are made for patients with symptoms of mandibular dysfunction or to prevent tooth wear caused by attrition. The common symptoms of mandibular dysfunction are:

Clicking on opening and closing the jaws.

Pain localized around the condyles, often starting in the morning and gradually increasing in severity during the day or occurring at any time without any associated factors.

Teeth are vaguely tender to bite upon early in the morning, indicating that clenching has occurred during the night.

Pain around the temporomandibular joint or associated with the muscles of mastication.

Difficult to manipulate the mandible in lateral excursions.

Occasionally, neck pain.

The Michigan splint is made to cover all standing teeth in the maxilla, with a canine rise to provide guidance in lateral excursions with posterior disclusion (see Fig. 5.2). If the splint relieves the symptoms, this may be diagnostic of mandibular dysfunction.

---

as an indication for treatment, especially if there is a history of repeatedly fracturing teeth. It is not known why some patients develop drifting teeth after extractions whereas, in others, no tooth movement occurs. Due to the complex relationship of the upper and lower teeth, it would be extremely useful to mount accurate study models on an adjustable articulator using a face-bow and a retruded contact jaw relation record in order to examine fully the occlusion and articulation.

What are the options for treatment?

Monitor the situation and patch or replace the restorations when necessary.

Re-organize the occlusion by placing crowns on posterior teeth, so eliminating occlusal interferences and restoring an ideal occlusal plane.

Use conventional orthodontic treatment to re-align the teeth before restoring and replacing teeth with crowns and bridges.

Use a Dahl-type appliance to reposition teeth.

● Monitoring

The simplest treatment would be to patch the fractured parts of the teeth with a material such as a glass ionomer and manage each situation as it arises. For teeth with more extensive restorations, individual crowns could be made to the existing occlusal relationship. Some patients may accept this treatment, but for others the potential for more frequent tooth restorations is unacceptable and so a more definitive treatment is preferable.

● Posterior crowns

Reducing the coronal height of the tilted upper molar can restore the occlusal plane and provide sufficient space for

a crown on the mesially drifted lower molar. However, the amount of over-eruption that has taken place is considerable and so the extent of reduction needed to ideally restore the tooth could result in devitalization of the pulp. Providing a crown on the lower molar is relatively straightforward, but in attempting to restore the occlusal plane the life-expectancy of the upper molar might be reduced.

Conformative occlusion

In this case, the simplest approach would be to make the occlusal morphology of the crowns conform to the existing intercuspal position. This accepts the existing vertical dimension of occlusion, any slide that exists between the retruded contact position and intercuspal position and the anterior guidance.

Re-organized approach

The alternative is to re-organize the occlusion completely. This is usually done when it is considered more convenient to establish a new occlusal position and articulation because there is no usable, existing intercuspal position. Because of its reproducibility, the retruded contact position is used as a treatment position (i.e. the intercuspal position is made coincident with the retruded contact position).

Recording the retruded contact position requires the mandible to be manipulated around its terminal hinge axis. It is often found, however, that such manipulation meets with great resistance from the muscles of mastication, particularly if there is muscle spasm, which forces the mandible to close into a protrusive position. If the mandible is resistant to manipulation around the terminal hinge axis, either a conformative approach can be accepted or an attempt made to relax the muscles sufficient to allow jaw manipulation and registration of the retruded contact position. To induce muscle relaxation, an anterior jig can be fitted to the incisal edges of the maxillary incisors, preventing tooth contact between the upper and lower arches. After 15–30 minutes the jig is removed and the jaw should be easier to manipulate. It has been argued that keeping the upper and lower teeth separated for this period of time breaks the cycle of proprioceptive feedback that returns the closing jaw into a protrusive position. Once the retruded contact position has been identified and recorded, a decision has to be made as to whether or not it is feasible and desirable to adjust the occlusal contacts so that the new intercuspal position is made coincident with the retruded position.

● Orthodontics

As previously described, the use of conventional cast restorations to 'upright' tilted teeth or to 'intrude' over-erupted teeth can be extremely destructive of tooth tissue and lead to pulp necrosis. In selected cases it might be possible to use fixed orthodontic appliance therapy to move malpositioned teeth. This type of treatment can be very prolonged, particularly in the adult patient, and so its success is in part dependent upon good patient compliance as well as technical issues such as adequate anchorage. Where orthodontics is possible, however, its application can make the difference between success and failure.

● Dahl appliance

A fixed metal or composite plate could be fitted to the lower molar and premolar teeth to intrude the upper molar. A fixed movable bridge or single implant could then replace the missing lower tooth. However, this would not address the mesial tilt of the lower molar.

What types of articulator are available?

Hand-located models.
Hinge.
Average value.
Semi-adjustable.
Fully adjustable.

For single crowns in a canine-guided occlusion, hand-held models may be adequate. For group function, cross bites and other malocclusions, the use of a semi-adjustable articulator with a face-bow transfer is highly desirable.

● Hand-located models

Often these are acceptable for individual crowns when the intercuspal position is easily located. If it is difficult to locate opposing casts accurately, there is great potential for crowns to be made with an incorrect occlusion. 'High' crowns will require chairside occlusal adjustment.

In this present case, considering the number of teeth needing restorations, hand-located models would not be sufficiently accurate. If they are used, the dentist must expect to spend some time adjusting the occlusal surfaces of the crowns to make them conform to the existing occlusal scheme. The major advantage of an articulator is that it reduces the time spent adjusting the crowns in the mouth. As articulators become more complex and the record of the position of the mandible gets more accurate, less time should be needed for intra-oral occlusal adjustment of new restorations.

● Simple hinge articulators

Provided there are sufficient teeth contacting in the intercuspal position, a hinge articulator may save clinical time. But when more than one crown is to be made or when the teeth to be prepared are involved in guiding movements, the hinge axis articulator becomes inaccurate.

In this present case, the canine is relatively prominent and so the occlusion is likely to be canine-guided. By definition, canine guidance causes the posterior teeth to separate at the very early stages of lateral mandibular excursive movement. As a consequence, the occlusal anatomy of the posterior teeth is not crucial as there is little risk that they will generate occlusal interferences. Conversely, if there is an absence of contact or small canine or incisor contact as, for instance, in an Angles class III or severe class II division 1 case, then the posterior teeth will inevitably form the guiding surfaces. It is in this type of situation that a semi- or fully adjustable articulator is required as these types are more able to reproduce jaw movement accurately.

● Average-value articulator

This is more accurate than the hinge articulator but less so than the semi-adjustable articulator. Therefore, using this type of articulator will reproduce some of the occlusal movements and consequently reduce the need for occlusal adjustment. The articulator is set up for the average person, with values fixed for the condylar guidance and intercondylar distance. The Bennett angle (the angle between the sagittal plane and the path of the advancing condyle during lateral mandibular movement) is fixed at 15°.

● Semi-adjustable articulators

These can be divided into arcon or non-arcon articulators. In a non-arcon articulator, such as the Dentatus ARH or ARL (AB Dentatus, Sweden) (Figs 5.3 and 5.4), the condylar ball is attached to the upper track, whereas in an arcon articulator the condyle is in the anatomically correct position on the lower track (Figs 5.5 and 5.6). Semi-adjustable articulators differ from the fully adjustable types by having a smaller range of adjustments available at, primarily, the condylar assembly. In particular, the intercondylar distance is usually fixed and the condylar path and Bennett angle is usually straight or set at 15°.

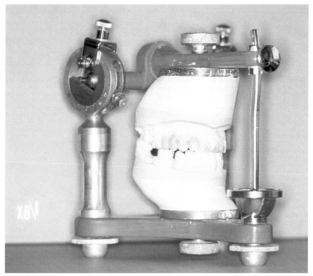

Fig. 5.3 The Dentatus ARH is a non-arcon articulator. The robust design means that it is not as susceptible to damage as others.

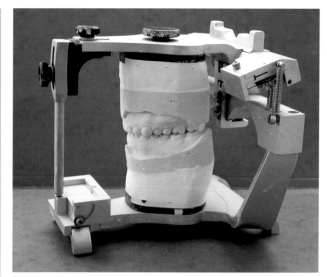

Fig. 5.5 The Denar articulator is an arcon type, with the condylar track on the upper member and the condyles on the lower member.

In this present case, as a number of teeth are being restored, a semi-adjustable articulator is the most convenient choice. A face-bow relates the spatial position of the maxilla to the condylar axis and Frankfort plane. Firstly, this ensures that the arc of opening and closing of the mandible is replicated on the articulator. This has the advantage that changes in the vertical dimension that will occur during mandibular excursive movements, as well as reconstructions at an increased vertical dimension, will be accurately replicated. Secondly, relating the maxillary position to the Frankfort plane gives an indication on the articulator of the position of the occlusal plane.

The general indications for using semi-adjustable articulators are shown in Box 5.2.

● Fully adjustable articulators

These can accurately reproduce all movements of the mandible. They need only be used rarely and in situations where occlusions are characterized by group function guidance, shallow condylar guidance angles and a significant immediate side-shift (Bennett movement). The adjustments available include:

The intercondylar distance.
The Bennett movement and angle.
The condylar shape and path.
Anterior guidance tables.
Adjustable to all right and left lateral records.

'Programming' a fully adjustable articulator requires the transfer of complex records of mandibular movement. These records are made by extra-oral tracing devices, such as the Pantograph or its electronic equivalent, the Pantronic.

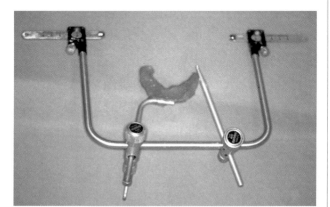

Fig. 5.4 The face-bow of the Dentatus ARH. Recording is more difficult than with the Denar slidematic face-bow. The hinge axis is estimated by positioning the face-bow 12–13 mm from the tragus along the ala–tragus line. Other face-bows use the external auditory meatus as the reference point and so are much easier to use.

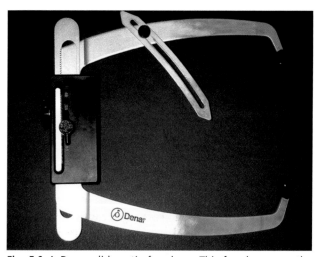

Fig. 5.6 A Denar slidematic face-bow. This face-bow uses the external auditory meatus to locate the hinge axis.

Box 5.2 General indications for using semi-adjustable articulators

If sufficient occlusal surfaces of teeth remain in contact after preparation and the intercuspal position can be easily recorded, there may be no need to use an articulator. If, however, the intercuspal position is lost after preparation or insufficient teeth remain, an occlusal record with a face-bow transfer is needed prior to treatment.

Patients with a class II division 1 incisal relationship have proclined upper anterior teeth; thus crowns made on these teeth are relatively simple and do not need an articulator. Conversely, crowns on the molar teeth, which are likely to be involved with group function during mandibular movements, are more complex; it is therefore important to achieve the optimum occlusal form, and an articulator is needed.

Crowns on posterior teeth for patients with a class II division 2 incisal relationship and who have retroclined anterior teeth are relatively straightforward as generally the canine guides the mandible in lateral excursions and the posterior teeth disclude early in the guidance. However, for anterior teeth, the situation is more complex as there is often little interocclusal space. An articulator is therefore helpful in the manufacture of the crowns as it will reduce the amount of chairside reduction and adjustment needed to ensure that the crown or restoration is placed comfortably.

Occasionally, when most of the occlusal surfaces of the teeth are being restored, the last standing teeth on one side can be left unrestored so that the existing interocclusal relationship remains and can be recorded. After the new crowns are fitted, the last standing tooth can be crowned.

Definitions of occlusal positions

● Static occlusal positions

Intercuspal position

The position of the mandible when there is the maximum contact and interdigitation between the upper and lower teeth.

Retruded contact position

This is the most reproducible position of the mandible and a commonly used reference point when re-organizing the occlusion. It is defined as the most retruded position of the mandible when the teeth are at first contact.

● Mandibular movements

Anterior guidance

In an Angles class I or class II division 2 occlusion, protrusion of the mandible is 'guided' by contact of the incisal edges of the mandibular anterior teeth against the palatal surfaces of the upper anterior teeth. In Angles class III and severe class II division 1 occlusions, the upper and lower anterior teeth do not contact each other during mandibular protrusion (Fig. 5.7). In these instances, it is cuspal inclines on the posterior teeth that provide the guiding surfaces. A very reduced or absent anterior guidance can severely complicate the provision of posterior tooth restorations as the shape and position of cusps and fossae become so much more critical.

Conversely, the fabrication of anterior restorations requires greater precision the deeper the anterior overbite becomes. For instance, in patients with a class II division 2 incisor relationship, the horizontal space between the upper and lower anterior teeth is very restricted. Anterior guidance comes into effect almost

immediately upon mandibular protrusion, causing the occlusal surfaces of the posterior teeth to disclude. Where possible, when making new crowns or bridges for someone with a class II division 2 incisal relationship, it is convenient to copy the existing anterior guidance. This is achieved by using a custom-made incisal guidance table (Fig. 5.8). Pre-operative study models are mounted on an articulator using an accurate face-bow and jaw-relation record. On the articulator's incisal table, laboratory acrylic or composite resin is used in combination with the incisal pin to construct a jig that replicates precisely the shape of the guidance provided by the existing anterior dentition. By using the jig, the palatal surfaces of the new anterior crowns or bridges can be designed to conform to the shape of the pre-existing dentition. This reduces the risk of introducing interferences that might result in signs of occlusal

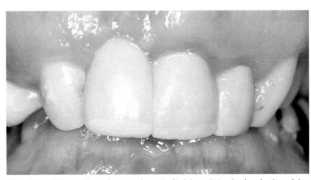

Fig. 5.7 This patient has a class II division 2 incisal relationship. Making crowns on the upper or lower anterior teeth is difficult. The situation is easier on the molars as canine guidance usually results in early disclusion of the molar teeth, meaning that the occlusal morphology is not so important.

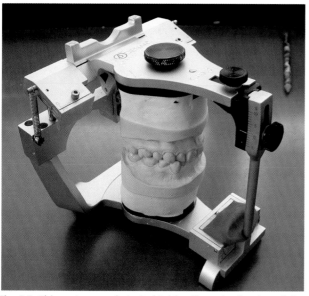

(a)

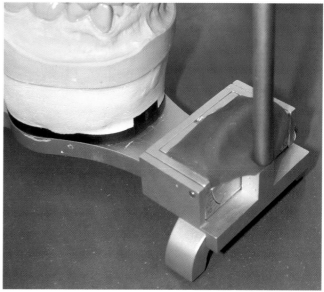

(b)

Fig. 5.8 This custom-made incisal table allows duplication of the anterior guidance of the existing restorations, or diagnostic wax-up to be copied on the definitive restorations.

trauma, such as tooth drifting or excessive loading of endodontically treated teeth.

For a patient with a class II division 1 incisal relationship, there may be no anterior guidance, especially with an anterior open bite, so protrusion is guided by the occlusal surfaces of the molars or premolars (Fig. 5.9).

Lateral excursions

For most people, the palatal contour of the upper canines guides the mandible in lateral movements when the teeth are in contact. This is called canine guidance. When more than one posterior tooth is involved, the process is called group function. For patients with class II division 1 incisal relationship, perhaps with an anterior open bite, guidance is carried by the premolar and molar teeth.

The side to which the mandible moves is called the working side; the opposite side is the non-working side. Contacts on the non-working side during lateral excursions are called non-working side interferences.

Occlusal interferences

An interference is defined as a contact occurring during an excursion which interferes with the free movement of the mandible. Often the interference develops as a result of dental treatment; for example, after a tooth is extracted, adjacent teeth may drift into new positions and interfere with the free sliding movement of the mandible (see Fig. 5.1). Normally, patients accommodate to the interference to such an extent that it is difficult to detect.

Fig. 5.9 This patient has an anterior open bite (class II division 1), so making crowns on the incisors on the right side is relatively straightforward. The right canine appears to be missing; therefore the premolars and molars will guide the mandible in lateral excursions. If crowns were needed on these teeth, the shape of their occlusal surface would be very important in order to maintain the existing occlusal relationship.

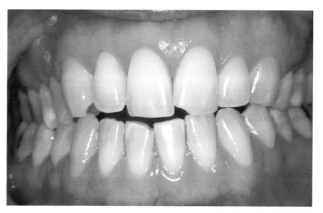

Occlusal stability

In some patients, the adjacent teeth remain in the same position following extractions and drifting does not occur. This is called a stable occlusion. When drifting of teeth does occur (e.g. after extractions), interferences may be introduced and the term unstable occlusion is used.

Occlusal vertical dimension

This is the vertical relationship between the maxilla and the mandible when the teeth are in the intercuspal position. This can be conveniently measured by marking dots on the skin above and below the lips and recording the distance between them. The freeway space is the distance between the upper and lower teeth when the mandible is relaxed.

Learning outcomes

- Management of over-erupted teeth.
- Definitions associated with occlusion.
- Choosing articulators.
- How to make a Michigan splint.

6

Managing worn teeth with composites

Clinical details

A 50-year-old man presents to you complaining about his worn teeth and would like the appearance improved (Fig. 6.1). He complains of regurgitation every day but has not sought medical advice; otherwise, there are no medical complications. His major concern is the appearance of the upper anterior teeth; the lower teeth do not show during normal function. The patient does not have dentinal sensitivity and there is no history of tooth grinding or clenching. What special tests might you consider and what is the cause of the tooth wear? What are the options to restore worn teeth and what restorative options are suitable for this patient? What complicating factors might you incur?

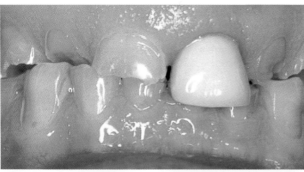

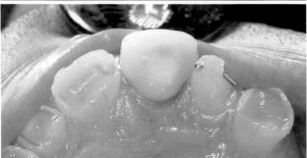

Fig. 6.1 This patient would like the appearance of his teeth improved.

Clinical observations

- Dentine is exposed on most upper anterior surfaces.
- He is partially dentate posteriorly.
- The posterior teeth that are present are moderately restored.
- There is no apparent loss of vertical dimension.
- The upper anterior crown was placed 15 years ago when the teeth were at the same incisal length.
- The palatal surfaces of the teeth are unstained.

What are the potential complicating factors?

The tooth wear has produced short clinical crowns without loss of vertical dimension. There has been some alveolar compensation. If conventional preparations for crowns were cut on the incisors and canines, there would be insufficient retention.

The tooth wear is extensive, exposing dentine but not involving the pulp. The upper left and right lateral incisors are particularly worn, with the exposure of secondary dentine.

The surface stain on the teeth can give an indication of the activity of the aetiology. In this case, the surfaces were clean and unstained, indicating that the source of the tooth wear was active. As soon as dietary stains form on the teeth they are removed by dietary or gastric acids. In cases where the surfaces are stained, this often means that the cause of the erosion is inactive as there is sufficient time for the tooth surfaces to take up dietary stains.

The buccal surface of the upper right lateral incisor does not contact the opposing tooth, indicating that erosion is a factor in the aetiology. The interdigitation of the other teeth and the wear from the porcelain crown on the lower incisors indicate that attrition is also an important component.

What special tests might be used?

Radiographic examination and vitality tests.
Tests for reflux.
Diagnostic casts.

● Radiographic examination and vitality tests

The periapical status of the upper teeth needs evaluating, as does the vitality of the worn teeth. There may be some suspicion of the vitality of the upper left lateral incisor, but it responded positively to an electric pulp test. There were no periapical changes visible on the radiographs.

● Tests for reflux

The pattern of wear on the upper incisors, together with the history of regurgitation, suggests that the aetiology is multifactorial, with regurgitation erosion and attrition as the major causes. To confirm the role of regurgitation, the patient could be referred for investigations by a gastroenterologist (see Box 6.1).

Box 6.1 Causes of tooth wear

Erosion

Teeth can be dissolved by acids found in the diet or from voluntary or involuntary regurgitation of stomach juice into the mouth, or, very rarely these days, from certain industrial processes. The pattern and distribution of erosion can be used to identify the origin of the acid.

Dietary erosion

Dietary acids can cause erosion in some patients (Fig. 6.2).

It is not necessarily the pH of a food or drink that is the most important factor in erosion; the titratable acidity is probably more important. The titratable acidity is the amount of alkali needed to neutralize the acid; the pH is a measure of the free hydrogen ions in solution. Generally speaking, most clinicians consider that titratable acidity is more important than pH. Some drinks have a relatively low pH but weak titratable acidity. Lemon and grapefruit juices are particularly erosive because they have a high titratable acidity, whereas some cola drinks are much less erosive.

Not only is the acidity of the drink important but also the way in which it is consumed; thus drinking habits are important as well as the duration of acid exposure. If someone swills or holds a drink in the palatal vault before swallowing, the acid remains in contact with the teeth for longer, thereby increasing the chance of erosion. Also, if the drink is taken with small sips over a long period of time, exposure to the acid is also increased. Young children are commonly seen holding or swilling carbonated drinks in their palate before swallowing. The extended exposure to acid is believed to result in the potential for more erosion.

Some patients change their dietary habits, especially after life-changing events. For instance, someone leaving home to go to university may have a significant change in lifestyle and consequently change their diet. It is important to investigate if the erosion is historical.

Gastric juice

Another common and destructive cause of erosion is regurgitation of gastric juice into the mouth. Eating disorders, such as anorexia, bulimia nervosa and rumination have all been recognized as causes of erosion, as has gastro-oesophageal reflux. Gastro-oesophageal reflux is the movement of gastric juice past and through the lower oesophageal sphincter; in some patients, this causes clinical symptoms, typically heartburn and epigastric pain. In susceptible patients, the reflux of the gastric juice reaches the mouth, when it is called regurgitation. Chronic alcoholism causes vomiting and gastro-oesophageal reflux, both of which will cause erosion (Figs 6.2 and 6.3).

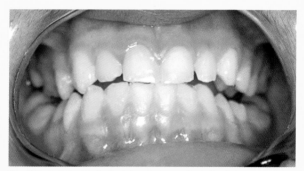

Fig. 6.2 Acidic drink first impacts against the buccal surfaces of the upper incisors (the lowers are generally protected by the lip) and causes erosion. If a drinking habit is present, such as holding or swilling prior to swallowing, the pattern of tooth wear may also involve the palatal surfaces.

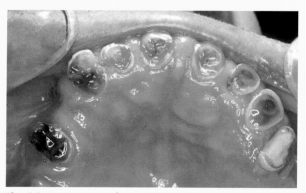

Fig. 6.3 Appearance of a patient with regurgitation erosion produced by a combination of reflux disease and chronic alcoholism.

Pattern of erosion

Acid originating from the stomach is thought to strike the palatal surfaces of the upper incisors, first eroding enamel, then, as the erosion progresses, the dentine is eventually involved. Theoretically, in the early stages of the process, the tongue protects the other surfaces of the teeth from the acid. As the erosive action persists, the protective mechanisms of the mouth are overwhelmed and a more generalized pattern of erosion occurs. Dietary acids tend to erode the labial surfaces of the anterior teeth as these are the first to contact the acid before it enters the oral cavity, where the acid is diluted and buffered by saliva. There is no universal consensus that palatal erosion is caused by stomach juice and that labial or buccal erosion is caused by the dietary acids; in severe cases, the distinction becomes less obvious.

Box 6.1 Causes of tooth wear—cont'd

Attrition

The wear of teeth by teeth is called attrition. It usually occurs in conjunction with erosion but also with abrasion. The teeth normally interdigitate and wear is equal in both arches. When the amount of wear is unequal the most likely cause is a combination of attrition and erosion. Attrition normally occurs in combination with bruxism, which is a parafunctional habit (Fig. 6.4).

Abrasion

Abrasion is the wear of teeth caused by surfaces other than teeth. Most commonly associated with tooth-brushing on the cervical margins of teeth, this lesion is usually caused by a combination of erosion, attrition, abrasion and possibly abfraction. The typical V-shaped lesion develops along the cervical margins of canines and premolars; it is less common around other teeth and rare on the palatal surfaces of teeth (Figs 6.4 and 6.5).

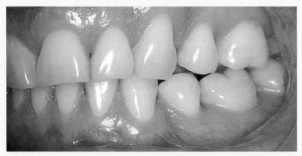

Fig. 6.4 Attrition is typically wear of tooth against tooth, with the severity being reasonably similar in both arches. Bimaxillary masseter hypertrophy is often clinically visible, supporting clinical diagnosis of parafunctional aetiology.

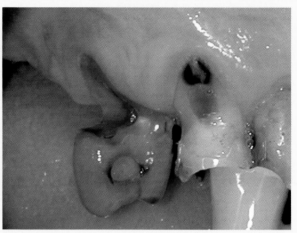

Fig. 6.5 Abrasion along the cervical margins of teeth. Traditionally, this has been associated with tooth-brushing, but it more likely to be multifactorial in nature, with erosion being a part of the aetiology.

Abfraction

There is some doubt as to whether this phenomenon is a theoretical or an actual process. In concept, minute stresses develop around the cervical margins of teeth as a result of the flexure of the root and the crown of the tooth. The cracks propagate from occlusal forces established along the tooth and from abrasion and erosion (Fig. 6.6).

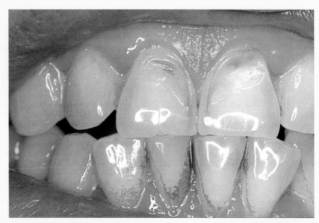

Fig. 6.6 Possibly an abfraction lesion or a combination of erosion, abrasion and attrition.

● Diagnostic casts

These can be helpful in planning the treatment or monitoring the tooth wear.

Diagnosis

The patient's tooth wear was caused by regurgitation erosion and a parafunctional habit causing attrition. The causes of tooth wear are described in Box 6.1. Sometimes it is not possible to determine the cause and, despite careful questioning, a definitive diagnosis cannot be made.

What are the options for treatment?

Monitoring.
Occlusal adjustment and restoration to the retruded contact position.
Full mouth rehabilitation.
Surgical crown lengthening.
Elective devitalization and post crowns.

● Monitoring

The most convenient and accurate way to assess the activity of tooth wear is to take study models of the patient's teeth and compare them to the teeth over relatively long periods of time. This process can continue over many years. Tooth wear is phasic in nature, with short periods of activity separated by longer periods of relative inactivity. During the longer inactive phase, tooth wear probably continues, but slowly. Provided the patient's main concern is the prevention of further wear to the teeth rather than an improvement in their appearance, monitoring is acceptable. However, it is imperative that the wear is monitored carefully rather than allowing the process to deteriorate to an extent where restorations become even more difficult (Figs 6.7 and 6.8).

In the present case, the symptoms of regurgitation and the clean and unstained tooth surfaces indicate that the tooth wear is active; treatment is therefore indicated.

● Occlusal adjustment

If the patient has a horizontal slide from the retruded contact position (RCP) to the intercuspal position (ICP), the adoption of RCP as the base position can be used to create space at the incisal edges of the upper anterior teeth. Adjustments to the occluding surfaces of the teeth are made until the RCP and ICP become coincident. A Michigan splint is helpful to determine the RCP, especially if manipulating the patient's mandible is difficult.

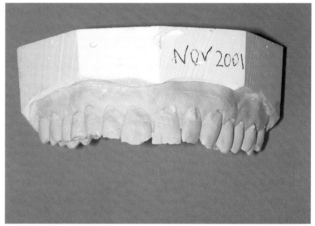

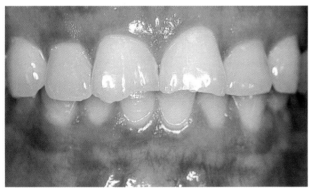

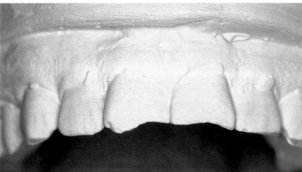

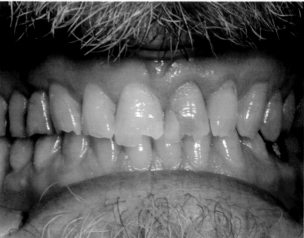

Fig. 6.7 The clinical photograph and the study model are of the same patient but taken about 8 years apart. There has been little tooth wear and, provided the patient is prepared to accept the appearance of the teeth, further monitoring would be indicated. (Courtesy Professor B. G. N. Smith).

Fig. 6.8 The study model of this patient was taken 8 months before the clinical photograph. It can be seen that the tooth wear has progressed, thus treatment is indicated to prevent further deterioration.

Once established, the RCP should be recorded and transferred to a semi-adjustable articulator. The sequence of tooth adjustments can be planned on the articulator and recorded in a step-by-step process until the RCP is the same as the ICP so that the same sequence can subsequently be used in the mouth.

● Full mouth rehabilitation

Restoring the occlusal surfaces of all standing teeth and increasing the occlusal vertical dimension will provide sufficient space for anterior restorations. Whilst increasing the vertical dimension in an edentulous patient might not be successful, the opposite is true for dentate patients. Increases in vertical dimension have traditionally been achieved in stages by using a bite-raising appliance to assess the patient's tolerance and thereafter restoring the teeth with crowns. However, the splints are often poorly tolerated and their use is questionable as they are often uncomfortable and delay the making of restorations at the new vertical dimension.

The Dahl appliance has been used more recently to allow localized movement of teeth to create space and has achieved widespread use in general practice. However, in this present case, there are relatively few occluding posterior teeth and use of a Dahl appliance is not possible. The recent improvement in bond strengths

of dentine-bonding agents has allowed composites to be used as short- to medium-term restorations rather than traditional crowns. The composites can be overlaid onto the posterior teeth to increase the vertical dimension and also added to the anterior teeth to improve their appearance. These restorations should be considered for the short to medium term to allow the new vertical dimension to be assessed and thereafter conventional crowns made.

It is a matter of judgement as to how much the vertical dimension should be increased, although in this case the incisal edge of the existing porcelain crown provides a convenient reference point. In principle, the new vertical dimension should be estimated from the original crown height. This is most conveniently achieved with a diagnostic wax-up. Sometimes, as in this case, an existing tooth or restoration gives a clue to the original position of the incisal edge and the new restorations are made to this position. However, when it is not possible to estimate the level of the unworn incisors from existing teeth or restorations, it may be useful to manipulate the patient into the RCP. The more retruded position creates vertical space between the incisors, which might be sufficient for the new restorations. Most patients will accept increases in the occlusal vertical dimension in the order of 2–4 mm. An advantage of using composites is that, if the increase is too large, the occlusion can be adjusted until a comfortable position is achieved.

● Surgical crown lengthening

The clinical crown height of teeth can be increased by surgically repositioning the gingival margin with alveolar bone recontouring (Fig. 6.9). This procedure creates longer teeth but maintains the existing vertical dimension. The teeth can then be prepared for crowns using conventional techniques.

Electrosurgery is contraindicated because this will only remove relatively small amounts of gingival tissue, and the amounts needed for increasing the clinical crown height would normally involve removal of bone. If the gingival margin is repositioned apically without bone removal, it will be able to return to its original location, resulting in subgingival margins and the potential for persistent gingival inflammation, which may eventually lead to uncontrolled recession.

The surgical procedure involves raising a surgical flap over the intended site and reducing the height and width of bone to increase the clinical crown height while maintaining the optimum distance of the alveolar bone to the gingival margin at about 3–4 mm. The gingival tissues are sutured apically. This exposes previously hidden vital dentine which may result in sensitivity. This can be managed with fluoride application, desensitizing toothpastes or the application of a dentine-bonding agent.

The eventual crown preparations should be finished on root dentine, which has a more oval cross-section

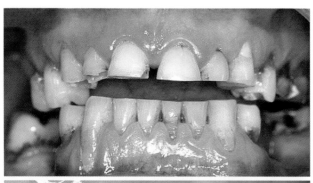
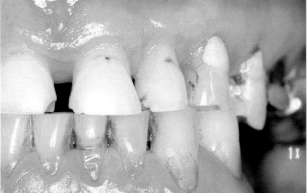

Fig. 6.9 Crown lengthening. The crown margin is surgically repositioned to a more apical position, so lengthening the crown height without changing the vertical dimension. This case shows crown lengthening and the results of successful periodontal treatment to control disease progression.

Box 6.2 Indications for the treatment of worn teeth

Patients' desire to improve their appearance

Intractable sensitivity

Loss of incisal edge

Uncontrolled tooth wear

than the coronal part of the tooth; the resulting crowns tend to be narrower at the gingival margin producing a more triangular appearance. Despite the increase in clinical crown height, a potential for pulpal exposure remains because tooth reduction is required to provide sufficient interocclusal space for crowns on the teeth where dentine is exposed on the palatal surfaces. Another potential disadvantage is that the peak of the interdental papilla may be lost following the surgical procedure and the normal contour of the gingival papilla can be compromised.

The timing of the placement of crowns is controversial. Some clinicians prefer placing crowns once the gingival tissues have fully recontoured after the surgery; this can take up to 6 months. Others prefer to prepare the teeth for crowns within days after the surgery, to prevent rebound of gingival tissues in a coronal direction. A compromise is to place provisional crowns within a week of the surgery and the definitive crowns nearer the 6-month period.

● Elective devitalization and post crowns

This procedure is not conservative and may reduce the prognosis of the teeth, but on occasions it is the only option available. Posts provide retention for the crowns but in doing so weaken the tooth and increase the potential for root fracture, which is further increased if the patient has a parafunctional habit.

The treatment for this patient

The activity of the tooth wear and the patient's preference for an improved appearance indicated that restorations were the appropriate treatment (indications for restorations for worn teeth are given in Box 6.2).

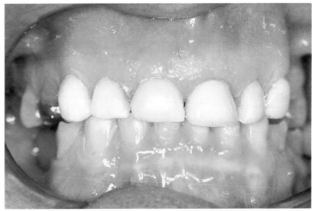

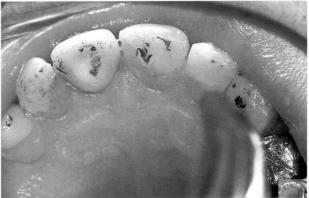

Fig. 6.10 This patient had composites placed on the anterior worn teeth and to the occlusal surfaces of the posterior teeth to increase the vertical dimension. The restorations were accepted by the patient as a medium-term solution; in the future, the crowns can be reduced to cores to retain conventional crowns. Articulating paper has been used to ensure that the anterior guidance is shared by the composite restorations and the existing porcelain crown.

Composites were chosen as interim restorations prior to crowns; in effect, they acted as intra-oral diagnostic wax-ups (Fig. 6.10). If needed, conventional crowns can be prepared later using the composites as cores.

Learning outcomes

- Using study casts to monitor tooth wear.
- Management of tooth wear.
- Understanding the concepts of surgical crown lengthening and the short clinical crown.
- Diagnosis and causes of tooth wear.

7

Dahl appliances

The patient is a 55-year-old man who has recognized that his teeth are getting shorter (Fig. 7.1). The palatal surfaces of the upper teeth have been eroded by regurgitated gastric acid over many years. He would like their appearance improved. The diagnosis of the wear is regurgitation erosion from chronic reflux disease; he is taking proton pump inhibitors to control his symptoms. What are the options to restore the appearance of his anterior teeth?

Clinical observations

- All the teeth are vital, there is no active decay and his remaining teeth are minimally restored.
- All anterior teeth gave a vital response to the electric pulp tester.
- The periodontal condition is under control.

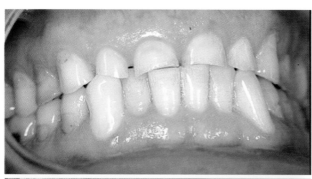

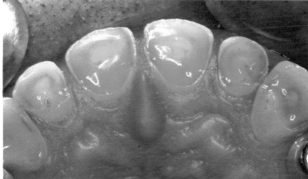

Fig. 7.1 Patient with regurgitation erosion (Case 7).

- The teeth are short but there has been no reduction in the vertical dimension. The tooth wear has been compensated by alveolar growth.
- The gingival margins of the upper incisors are slightly lower (more incisal) than the canines.

What are the potential complicating factors?

Short clinical crowns.
The gingival margins.

● Short clinical crowns

The teeth have short clinical crowns and, if they were to be prepared conventionally, the extent of incisal reduction would leave insufficient clinical crown height to retain a conventionally cemented crown. Also, conventional preparations would probably expose the pulps of these teeth, necessitating endodontic treatments. Additional crown height is needed to provide adequate retention for conventionally luted crowns.

● The gingival margins

There is normally a step in the contour of the gingival margins between the canines and lateral incisors. In this case, this step is more pronounced and represents the effects of alveolar compensation (Fig. 7.2). As wear progresses on the palatal surfaces of the upper incisors, the upper and lower teeth continue to maintain contact through a process called alveolar compensation. If this is not reversed, the gingival margins of the eventual restorations will remain at the lower level.

What are the options for treatment?

Dahl appliance.
Occlusal adjustment.
Full mouth rehabilitation.
Surgical crown lengthening.

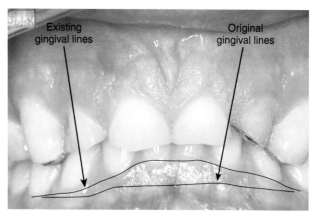

Fig. 7.2 Alveolar compensation has occurred in this patient after tooth wear on the palatal surfaces of the upper incisor teeth. The lower teeth have moved towards the occlusal plane by an increase in height of alveolar bone around the lower incisors. This results in short clinical crowns without any space available for conventional crowns; space therefore needs to be created.

Dahl appliance

This appliance is usually cemented to worn teeth and, by a combination of intrusion and extrusion, provides the vertical space needed to prepare conventional crowns. The original appliance described by Dahl used a removable appliance, but a fixed one is more commonly used. The occluding surface should be flat so that the forces applied by the lower incisors pass along the long axis of the upper anterior teeth.

Restoring in a more retruded position

If the patient is positioned into the retruded contact position (RCP), this posterior and superior movement can create anterior space. Once the RCP is identified, occlusal adjustment is needed on the occluding teeth to make the RCP and intercuspal position coincident. In principle this process might appear simple but it is not and can be quite destructive of tooth tissue.

Full mouth rehabilitation

If the patient is partially dentate, a Dahl appliance might not be effective. The intrusive and extrusive movement needed to create the vertical space is dependent upon the presence of sufficient teeth. If too many teeth are missing, the opposing forces cannot be established and so no vertical movement occurs. Alternatively, vertical height can be created by placing crowns on all occluding teeth, thereby increasing the vertical dimension; this is called a full mouth rehabilitation. Since the interocclusal height has been increased, there is no need for incisal reduction, leaving sufficient crown height for conventional preparations. The indications for increasing the occlusal vertical dimension for restoring teeth are listed in Box 7.1.

Surgical crown lengthening

Surgical crown lengthening involves repositioning the gingival margin apical to their existing position. The gingival tissues are surgically retracted and sufficient height and width of alveolar bone is removed to lengthen the clinical crown height. It is an uncomfortable procedure which can be poorly tolerated without sedation and good local anaesthesia. Surgical crown lengthening is usually indicated in partially dentate patients.

Box 7.1 Indications for increasing the occlusal vertical dimension

Reduced vertical dimension of occlusion following tooth loss.

Short teeth as a result of tooth wear.

Multiple occlusal interferences as a consequence of tooth loss and drifting.

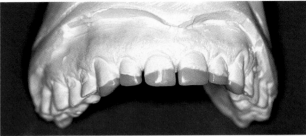

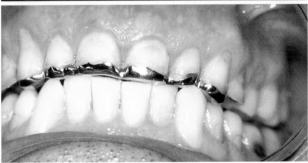

Fig. 7.3 A diagnostic wax-up used to assess the length of the restorations and the eventual Dahl appliance cemented onto the upper incisors. The Dahl is placed where the wear had occurred and provides vertical space through a combination of extrusion and intrusion.

What is a Dahl appliance?

An anterior Dahl appliance creates vertical space by inducing the posterior teeth to over-erupt (about 60% of the movement), together with some intrusion of the opposing teeth (about 40% of the movement). Dahl appliances need a virtually intact dentition to allow the intrusion/extrusion movement to occur. They can be removable or cemented to the teeth, but they tend to be better tolerated when they are fixed to the teeth.

Assessing the length of the restorations

The first stage is to assess the crown height of the restorations. Clinically, by manipulating the patient into

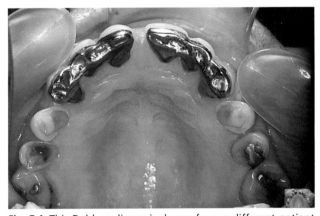

Fig. 7.4 This Dahl appliance is shown from a different patient where the indentations are placed on the palatal surfaces. The steps correspond to the intercuspal position of the lower incisors. These surfaces should be made flat so that the force of the lower incisors is directed along the vertical axis of the teeth.

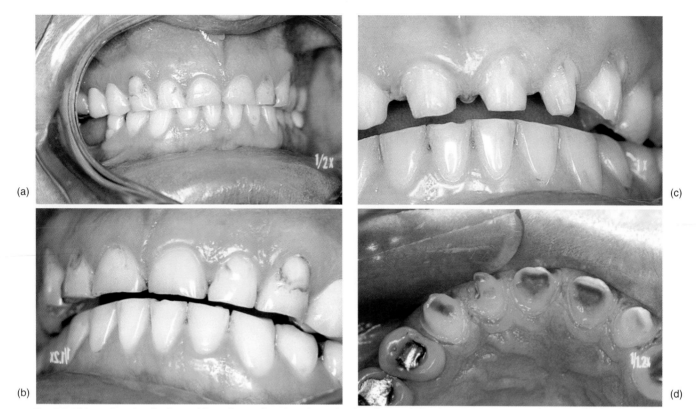

Fig. 7.5 This patient has had a Dahl appliance fitted to the palatal surfaces of the shortened upper anterior teeth (a). By a process of intrusion/extrusion, vertical space was created, eliminating the need for incisal and palatal reduction for metal ceramic crowns (b). The eventual preparations are of optimum length (c) and preserve the vitality of the tooth because the palatal surfaces remain unprepared (d).

RCP it may be possible to identify posterior contacts which give an indication of the original vertical relationship prior to the wear. In some cases it is not possible to do this, but the technician still needs to know the height of the restorations. A diagnostic wax-up mounted on a semi-adjustable articulator will give an indication of the proposed increase in clinical crown height (Fig. 7.3). If the models are mounted on the articulator in the intercuspal position using a face-bow recording, the relationship of the teeth in the upper and lower arches can be assessed. The most important step is to assess by how much to raise the incisal pin and so increase the occlusal vertical dimension. Normally, this can be estimated from a diagnostic wax-up, which provides the ideal anterior crown height. The increase in the crown height should be matched to provide the optimum appearance.

The Dahl appliance should be designed so that opposing forces from the teeth are directed along the long axis of the teeth (Fig. 7.4). If the force is directed buccally, there is a potential for an orthodontic movement of the linked anterior teeth in a labial direction, leaving gaps distal to the canines. The appliance should be cemented with a lute that will allow easy removal (e.g. Poly F; DeTrey Surrey, UK) or a glass ionomer. The length of time needed to produce the necessary movements will be individual to each patient. However, normally, the bigger the increase the quicker the movement.

Once the Dahl appliance is removed the teeth can be prepared for conventional crowns, eliminating the need for further reduction of the teeth.

Alternative approaches

There is no reason why a direct or indirect composite cannot be used as the appliance; this would improve its appearance. A directly placed composite with the appropriately placed indentations would be time-consuming.

The definitive crowns could have the Dahl appliance made onto the palatal surfaces. This produces the same result as a Dahl appliance but with a better appearance. Once the movement has occurred, the steps in the crowns could be removed and the surfaces polished.

Tooth preparations at the existing occlusal vertical dimension might produce sufficient crown height to adhesively bond the restorations.

● The preparations

Once the Dahl appliance has created sufficient vertical space, the teeth are prepared using conventional principles of retention (Fig. 7.5). The advantage of the Dahl appliance is that the space is created where the wear originally occurred so there is no need for any palatal reduction which preserves the vitality of the teeth. An interocclusal record is taken and the information sent to the laboratory where the crowns are made to prescription.

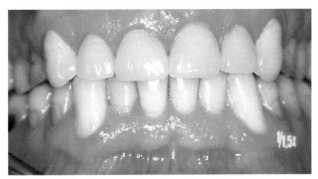

Fig. 7.6 The final crowns from Case 7 after the Dahl appliance was removed.

● The crowns

The crowns are made to the same shape as predicted in the diagnostic wax-up. Note how much movement of the posterior teeth has occurred, resulting in the closure of the gap (Fig. 7.6).

Learning outcomes

- ● Assessing worn teeth.
- ● Management of worn teeth using Dahl appliances.
- ● Reasons for increasing the occlusal vertical dimension for restorations.

8

Broken-down molars

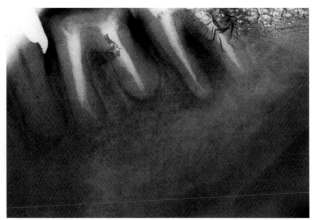

Fig. 8.2 The radiographic appearance of the re-root-treatments of the patient in Case 8.

Clinical details

A colleague has asked you to restore the worn teeth of a 20-year-old woman who suffers from bulimia nervosa (Fig. 8.1). The eating disorder at the time of presentation was under control and was not a significant factor in her management; there were no other medical problems. Her molars had been originally root-treated 2 years ago due to intractable sensitivity, but the practitioner had overfilled the canals and perforated the apex. Six months ago the tooth was re-root-treated and since that time the tooth has remained symptomless (Fig. 8.2). She would now like crowns to restore shape and function. How could you restore the patient's molars and what problems might you envisage? How long do you normally wait until commencing post preparations in root-treated teeth?

Clinical observations

■ The lower first molar has been re-root-treated but the root is shortened due to resorption.
■ There is no coronal seal.
■ Alveolar compensation has produced insufficient interocclusal space for conventional restorations.
■ There was no palatal dental erosion.

■ The molars on the contralateral side are equally worn.
■ The upper left premolar needs extracting.
■ The amalgam on the premolar had a distal overhang.

What are the potential complicating factors?

The alveolar bone and periodontal tissues on opposing teeth have compensated for the wear on the lower molars by moving towards the occlusal plane. The result is that there is very little coronal tissue available for crown preparations. Even if the teeth were extracted, there would be insufficient space for a partial denture.

The roots are short and posts will not provide sufficient retention for crowns. The resorption has complicated the situation and may compromise further management if the existing root treatments do not prevent the situation worsening.

The obturation of the root canals is satisfactory on both molars, but periapical radiolucencies remain associated with both teeth. In these circumstances, treatment is usually delayed until there is radiographic evidence of healing. The absence of a coronal seal may contribute to the slow healing around the periapical tissues, and a better seal should be placed before further treatment is commenced. However, since the tooth has already been re-root-treated, further treatment is not

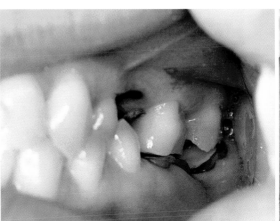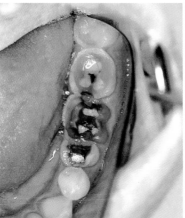

Fig. 8.1 The appearance of the teeth of the patient in Case 8.

> **Box 8.1** Dentine-bonding agents
>
> Modern dentine-bonding agents have bond strengths between composite and dentine that approach the strength of the bond between enamel and composite. Dentine is partly organic and comprises a relatively wet surface formed from fluid transport along the dentinal tubules. Composites, on the other hand, are hydrophobic. Therefore, dentine-bonding agents need to link a wet to a dry surface. Most accomplish this by using relatively low molecular weight fluids that flow into the tubules; these are subsequently strengthened by incorporating increasingly resinous materials. The materials gain strength mainly from micro-mechanical retention of the material within the dentinal tubules, but there is also a contribution from infiltration of the hybrid layer (Fig. 8.6). This porous layer forms after acid etching which is infiltrated with the dentine-bonding agent to create a hybrid layer. Some of the resin infiltrates the porous surface whilst the rest passes along the tubules to form dentine tags. The combination of an infiltrated hybrid layer and resin tags provides the retention of the material to dentine.
>
> Most materials require short etching times and longer washing times to obtain optimum bond strengths. The acid demineralizes the smear layer that is formed after cutting enamel or dentine. The layer is firmly attached to the tooth surface and, following etching, forms part of the hybrid layer. Newer dentine-bonding agents have eliminated the need to acid-etch the tooth separately and have combined the etching process within the same bottle as the bonding agent. Some manufacturers use weaker acids to disrupt the surface layer rather than remove it (e.g. Adper Prompt; ESPE, Germany). The concept of wet bonding reflects the mode of action of these materials. The low molecular weight enables a bond to be formed between the hydrophilic dentine and the hydrophobic composite; if the tooth is desiccated, the bond strengths achieved are not maximal.

indicated, but if the area failed to resolve, surgical intervention could be considered. In situations where an adequate root treatment has been completed, and there is little chance that it could be improved, any delay in placing a definitive coronal restoration is unnecessary.

When to restore root-treated teeth

There are no hard and fast rules about restoring root-treated teeth apart from perhaps the need to establish an effective coronal seal. Once this is achieved, the timing of placing posts is based on clinical experience. However, there are some guiding principles. For instance, if the obturation of the canals appears to be satisfactory and it is unlikely to be improved, post preparation and the definitive restoration could be placed almost immediately.

If obturation of the canal is not within 1–2 mm of the radiographic apex, post preparation immediately after obturation is not indicated and the tooth should be reviewed until the radiographic appearance indicates that resolution of the radiolucency is occurring. In this case, as a specialist has placed the root treatment and it is unlikely to be improved, the restoration can be commenced immediately.

What are the options for treatment?

Extract the teeth and, following bony recontouring, make a lower partial denture.

Cement a Dahl appliance on the worn teeth to produce axial movement and create space for restorations.

Replace coronal seals in the root-treated teeth and monitor tooth wear.

● Extraction

Removing the teeth might worsen the situation in a patient who has a recognized potential for tooth movement. If the teeth are extracted, the opposing teeth might continue to move towards the occlusal plane which, in this case, would be the alveolar ridge, making future restorations very difficult. The safest option would be to replace the coronal restorations and not change the vertical relationship. But this would not satisfy the patient's need for posterior crowns.

● Dahl appliance

The Dahl appliances can be made of metal, direct or indirect composites or even porcelain. The difference is that, when metal is selected, the laboratory technician creates the occlusal morphology of the tooth but, when direct composite is used, the clinician must do this. There is no reason why a Dahl appliance cannot be used on molars and, in this case, considering the extent of the problems associated with the molars, it was the only way

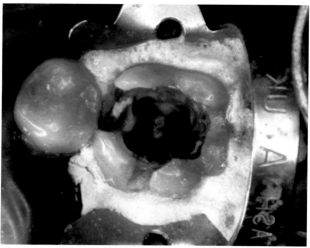

Fig. 8.3 Nayyar core. The gutta percha is removed 3–4 mm down the radicular canals over which is packed amalgam. The combination of the buccal walls and the root canals provide retention for the core.

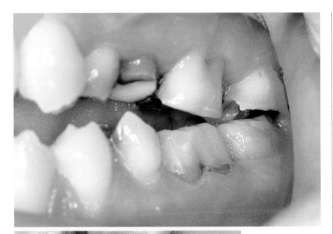

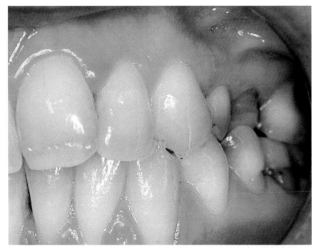

Fig. 8.5 About 8 months after the composites were placed, the teeth, by a combination of extrusion and intrusion, have re-organized themselves to a better occlusal plane, allowing the teeth to be restored with whatever material is appropriate.

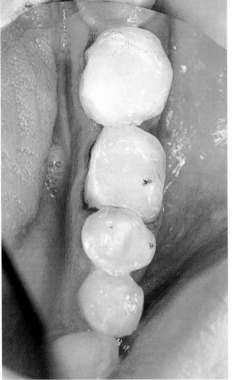

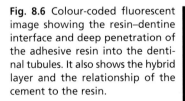

Fig. 8.4 Composites have been added to the occlusal surfaces of the molars and premolars to increase the vertical dimension by about 4 mm.

to create space. Direct composites were placed onto the tooth surface, linked with a dentine-bonding agent (see Box 8.1) and placed into the canals using the Nayyar core principle (Fig. 8.3). It is helpful to remember that, if you add 1 mm of composite onto the occlusal surface of a molar, the increase in height on the incisors is 3 mm. This ratio of 1:3 results from the incisors being further away from the axis of rotation (Fig. 8.4).

The orthodontic movement, by reversing the alveolar compensation, produces changes to the clinical crown height so that conventional or definitive restoration can be undertaken (Fig. 8.5).

Learning outcomes

- Management of a broken-down molar.
- How to use posterior Dahl appliances to increase vertical space.
- How dentine-bonding agents work.

Fig. 8.6 Colour-coded fluorescent image showing the resin–dentine interface and deep penetration of the adhesive resin into the dentinal tubules. It also shows the hybrid layer and the relationship of the cement to the resin.

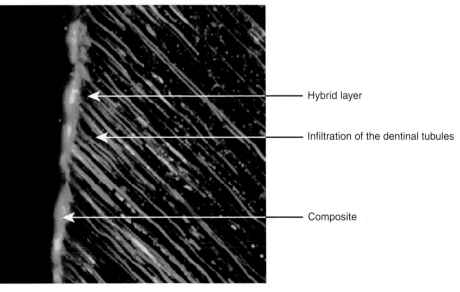

Hybrid layer

Infiltration of the dentinal tubules

Composite

9

Post crowns

Clinical details

A 55-year-old, medically fit, patient attends your surgery and during treatment you decide that you have to use post-retained crowns to restore the upper lateral incisors (Fig. 9.1). What factors do you consider when choosing a particular type of post and core?

Clinical observations

- The patient has a class I incisal relationship.
- The canines and central incisors are vital to the electric pulp tester.
- The patient's lip line is favourable and does not compromise the aesthetics of the eventual crowns.

What types of post are available?

Posts can be classified as either laboratory-made (indirect) or prefabricated (direct). The former are cast, with an inclusive core, from an impression taken of the prepared post canal. The latter are circular cross-section dowels, which are available in a range of materials that are cemented into the prepared post canal and to which are attached cores made from a plastic material, usually amalgam or composite.

How do you choose between a custom-made post and a prefabricated post?

There are no hard and fast rules and in many situations it is possible to use either type.

The main advantages of the custom-made post are that the core is an integral part of the casting and the shape of the post is made to fit the prepared post canal accurately. This is particularly significant when the root canal is oval in cross-section.

The main advantages of prefabricated posts are that they provide a single-visit solution to building up an endodontically treated tooth. Also, wrought metal posts are generally speaking stronger than cast posts for any given diameter.

In general terms, therefore, cast posts and cores are most suitable in situations where the post canal is wide (>1.25 mm), irregular in shape and there is little remaining coronal tooth tissue. Conversely, prefabricated posts are most appropriate when the post canal is narrow, circular in cross-section and some tooth tissue remains above the gingival margin.

Several dental product manufacturers supply comprehensive kits containing the armamentaria and components necessary either to prepare and construct custom-made posts or to install prefabricated posts. The kits contain post canal preparation drills in a range of diameters with size-matched impression, burn-out, temporary and wrought-metal prefabricated posts. Also available are kits for the installation of prefabricated 'aesthetic' posts made from materials such as fibre-reinforced composite resin or ceramic.

● Indirect (cast or custom-made) posts

Indirect posts are custom-made in the laboratory from an impression taken of a root canal prepared by a drill. Normally, the post drill, impression and the burn-out post are size-matched so that the cast post accurately fits the hole created by the post drill. But this need not be necessary. Cast posts can be made from tapered or parallel-sided post holes. They derive their retention from the close fit between the post and the root surface which, when combined with a cement lute, provides adequate retention for a crown.

● Direct (prefabricated) posts

There are a large variety of direct posts and perhaps the most convenient method of their classification is threaded and non-threaded. Direct posts gain their retention from ensuring that the post hole prepared by a drill is closely matched to the same-sized prefabricated post.

Non-threaded posts

Parallel-sided non-threaded posts are generally accepted to be one of the most retentive types of post and have been the mainstay of this type of system for many years (Figs 9.2–9.4). Normally, they are made of stainless steel or titanium, but more recently carbon fibre, composite

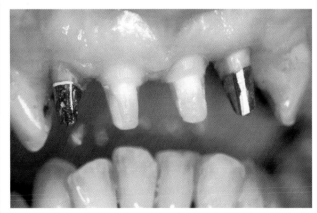

Fig. 9.1 The posts from the patient in Case 9. (Courtesy Dr David Ricketts.)

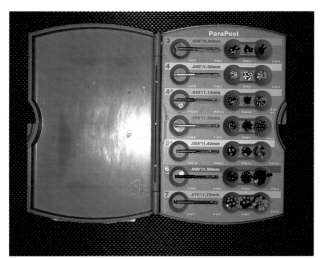

Fig. 9.2 A non-threaded post system (Coltene/Whaledent, Liechtenstein). The drill, temporary, burn-out and impression post are all size-matched and colour-coded to simplify the process.

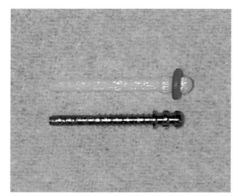

Fig. 9.4 The fibre white post (top) and the XT-threaded post, which has a passive fit at the apical part of the post and a threaded part towards the core (Coltene/Whaledent, Liechtenstein). The white post is suggested for anterior post crowns where it produces a better appearance than metal ones for all-ceramic crowns.

and ceramics have been used. One of the major criticisms of metal posts is their opacity, especially beneath all-ceramic crowns; a white or tooth-coloured post can reduce this effect and improve the translucency and appearance of the crown.

Non-threaded direct posts usually have serrations along the length of the post to improve the flow of cement during the luting phase. A number of manufacturers use colour-coded systems, which are size-matched for the drill, temporary post, the impression post, burn post and the direct post. Some manufacturers produce tapered posts designed to match the natural shape of the root canal; others have produced hybrids where the apical portion is parallel-sided and the coronal part is tapered.

Threaded systems

This type of post has received considerable criticism, not necessarily because of the concept but rather because of their clinical misuse. Similar to threading holes in metal, a thread needs to be tapped into the hard dentine surface of the root canal prior to screwing in the post. Why many threaded posts fail is that clinicians use them like wood screws, assuming that they are self-tapping; this creates cross-threading on the dentine surface, producing poor retention of the post and high stress concentration, leading to cracking of the dentine. Often the only area of contact is between the dentine and the outer edge of the thread along the post.

If the dentine is carefully prepared, threaded systems can be quite retentive. There are a number on the market, either parallel-sided or tapered (Fig. 9.5). Threaded posts can be particularly helpful in restoring fractured premolars where there is little coronal tissue remaining. Recently, one manufacturer introduced a tapered apical portion with a parallel-sided post, which is threaded coronally; they claim superior retention.

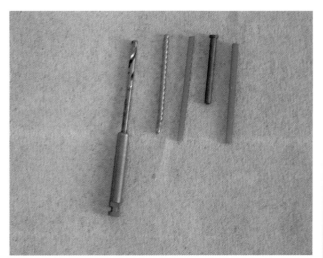

Fig. 9.3 The drill, stainless-steel direct, plastic burn-out, temporary and impression posts are all size-matched (Coltene/Whaledent, Liechtenstein). The burn-out post is used by the technician to make the cast post, which has a serrated surface.

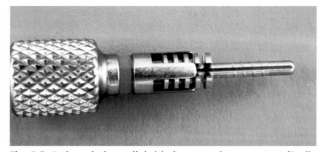

Fig. 9.5 A threaded parallel-sided post and core system (Radix Anchor; Dentsply, Weybridge, UK). The post has a series of drills, a post drill, a gutta percha removal bur, coronal preparation bur and the post itself, all colour- and size-matched.

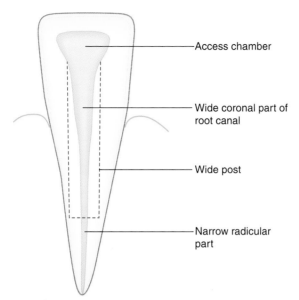

Fig. 9.6 If a post hole is tapered with a wide coronal area and narrower apical area, a direct post will only fit the part of the root surface that has been prepared by the post drill, usually in the apical third of the root (see Fig. 9.9). Therefore, a cast post that is custom-made to fit the post hole along all of its length will be superior to a direct post.

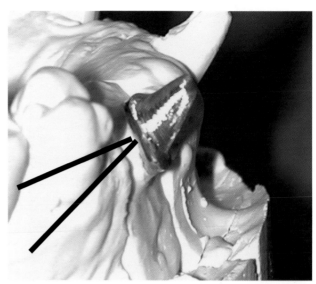

Fig. 9.7 The post angulation can be altered in cast posts, unlike prefabricated ones, which must follow the angulation of the root canal. The angle between the post and the core can be changed to produce a more convenient angulation for the crown.

● Comparison of direct and indirect posts

In most cases, the choice of a direct or indirect post relies on clinical judgement and experience. In the many studies that have compared the two techniques, little difference has been observed in their relative retentive capacities. There are some situations, however, where a cast post has advantages over a direct post:

> If a post hole is tapered with a wide coronal area and narrower apical area, direct posts will only fit the part of the root surface that has been prepared by the post drill, usually in the apical third of the root (Fig. 9.6). Therefore a cast post which is custom made to fit the post hole along all of its length will be superior to direct posts.
>
> Another advantage of cast posts is that the angulation of the core can be changed. The core on a direct post must be directly in line with the post. In a cast post, the core and the post can be made in slightly different directions to overcome differences in the angulation of the teeth (Fig. 9.7).
>
> Both cast and direct posts can fail. If the core and post are not made integrally, the core may become separated from the post, leading to loss of the restoration. Cast posts can fail around the core too, especially if there is a disparity in the size of the core to the post. After casting, a large core will tend to cool and solidify from its molten state more slowly than the thinner post. Pores can develop at the junction between the two, predisposing the metal to fracture.
>
> Many temporary posts are unstable and unretentive despite the best efforts of the manufacturers. Direct posts eliminate the need to use temporary posts and

enable the dentist to place a core immediately onto the newly cemented post and so provide a retentive temporary crown attached to the definite post.

The best way of ensuring success is to retain the maximum amount of dentine and the minimum diameter of post commensurate with the strength necessary to support the core.

Retrieval of posts

Provided a non-adhesive cement has been used, most posts can be retrieved from the canal. Ultrasonic instruments, with copious irrigation to prevent overheating, are invaluable for removing conventional cemented posts. The ultrasonic tip should be positioned onto the junction between the post and the tooth where the cement lute is visible and the ultrasound continued for as long as necessary. A shallow groove should be placed along the junction between the post and the tooth and the ultrasonic tip placed in this area. If an adhesive cement has been used, the chances of retrieval are reduced. The adhesive cement will remain along the root surface and be almost impossible to remove. This is especially important when considering using tooth-coloured posts that can be drilled out.

How can you test the vitality of the teeth?

Electric pulp test.
Cold stimulation.
Heat stimulation.

● Electric pulp test

This involves stimulating the nerve fibres in the pulp by passing an electric current through the tooth. The technique does not work on crowned teeth unless the tip of the probe can be placed onto visible dentine. Whilst the

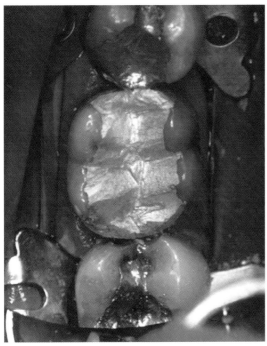

Fig. 9.8 The amalgam core provides support for a gold crown. A metal–ceramic crown preparation might remove the buccal wall of enamel and dentine. This might in turn remove a major part of the retention for the amalgam, resulting in the loss of the restoration.

technique cannot be considered accurate as it does not determine the pulp blood flow, it is the most reliable of the commonly used techniques.

● Cold stimulation

Usually, ethyl chloride is applied with a cotton-wool pledget to the labial surface of the tooth. This test does not always provide an accurate indication of the tooth's vitality since patients have different sensitivities to cold.

● Heat stimulation

Usually, a hot gutta percha stick is applied to elicit the sensation of heat. This test is rarely used since it is difficult to control the temperature.

What are your choices for core materials?

Amalgam.
Composite.
Glass ionomer.

● Amalgam

Many practitioners prefer amalgam as the choice for cores when using direct posts posteriorly (Fig. 9.8). Some manufacturers have produced fast-setting amalgams, which can be prepared within an hour, but in most cases the core must be prepared a day after placement. Amalgams may corrode which, in theory, produces by-products that reduce the gap size around the material/tooth interface and so reduce the amount of micro-leakage. The effect of newer high-copper products, which have a reduced gamma

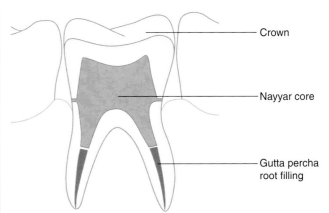

Fig. 9.9 Nayyar core. The principle of the Nayyar core is to gain retention from the coronal portion of the root canals. The gutta percha is removed with a non-end-cutting bur to a depth of 3–4 mm and the material, usually amalgam, is packed into the holes. Generally, this technique is most successful if there is additional support from any remaining cusps. It is less likely to succeed if the tooth is virtually de-coronated.

II phase and consequently less corrosion, is unknown. Amalgam without the use of adhesive bonding does not adhere to teeth and therefore additional forms of retention are needed, such as pins, grooves, slots and undercuts.

A Nayyar core can be used as an alternative to a post, especially when sufficient tooth structure is remaining (Fig. 9.9). Gutta percha is removed 3–4 mm along the coronal part of the root canal, just below the access chamber, into which is packed either composite or amalgam. The bulk of the material provides the support of the core. With either material, additional retention can be provided by using a dentine-bonding agent.

● Composite

Composites are the choice core materials for anterior teeth. Cores for posterior teeth can be made from amalgam or composite and the choice between the two is not critical.

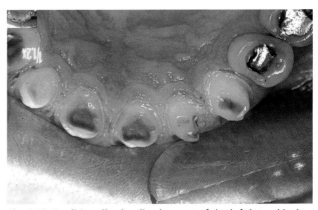

Fig. 9.10 Traditionally, the distal aspect of the left lateral incisor would be patched with a glass ionomer to make a conventional preparation shape. Alternatively, the crown could be made to the existing preparation shape and an adhesive cement used to retain the crown.

If a dentine-bonding agent is used to seal the material to the tooth, additional retention for the core will be gained. However, in deep cavities, the success of the bonding agent is less and the potential for a gap increases. The bond between composite, the dentine-bonding agent and the tooth is liable to failure and micro-leakage will occur as with any other material. Water will also be absorbed, which may affect dimensional stability. For these reasons, a number of clinicians prefer amalgam as a posterior core material.

● Glass ionomers

Whilst relatively useful for small additions to cores, the bond to dentine is not strong enough if the material becomes the major component of the core. However, small additions to cores become unnecessary if adhesive cement is used to cement the crown (Fig. 9.10). The crown can be made directly to the broken part of the tooth or restoration. If cement lute is not adhesive, adding to the core with glass ionomer is acceptable.

Learning outcomes

- ● To recognize types of posts.
- ● Principles of post retrieval.
- ● Vitality tests.
- ● Use of core materials.

10

Replacing canines

Clinical details

This 50-year-old lady presents to your surgery requesting a bridge to replace her denture (Fig. 10.1). She lost the tooth 1 year ago following trauma and managed to cope with an unretentive partial denture, but she would like a bridge. She smokes 10 cigarettes a day and has taken anti-hypertensive medication for 5 years; otherwise, her medical history is clear.

Clinical observations

- The space between the upper lateral incisor and premolar is 12 mm.
- The lower canine has over-erupted into the edentulous space.
- The upper right lateral incisor is unrestored, has a short clinical crown and is inclined mesially.
- The upper right premolars have extensive amalgams and are caries-free.
- The periodontal condition is good.
- She has a low lip line which hides the cervical margins of her teeth.
- There are no other dental problems.

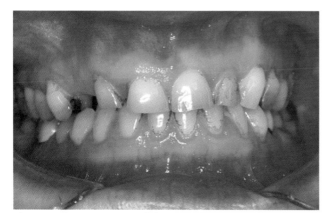

Fig. 10.1 The appearance of the patient in Case 10, showing the missing upper right canine.

What are the potential complicating factors?

Horizontal space.
Vertical space.
The lateral incisor has a short clinical crown.
Replacement of a canine.

● Horizontal space

The space between the upper first premolar and the lateral is longer than the average width of a canine (8 mm). A choice has to be made when making a bridge whether to accept the space and make a wide tooth pontic or to alter the width of the adjacent crowns. Asymmetry in the upper anterior region usually has a poor appearance and is poorly tolerated. Altering the width of the adjacent teeth with the crowns might mask this problem.

● Vertical space

The over-eruption of the lower canine will complicate treatment. The available space needs to be assessed on a semi-adjustable articulator together with an accurate diagnostic wax-up. It may be possible to position the pontic to a more pronounced buccal position and avoid any change to the vertical relationship of the teeth. If this is not possible, additional vertical space is needed to restore the edentulous area.

How can you create vertical space?

Restoring the patient to a more posterior and superior position. Usually, the most convenient position is the retruded contact position (RCP). In this case the RCP may not create sufficient space for a pontic.

Vertical space can be created with a Dahl appliance. A provisional bridge could be made with a flat occlusal plane, which would intrude the opposing canine and allow over-eruption of adjacent teeth; the space created would be sufficient to place a pontic in the ideal tooth position. The design of the pontic should include a flat surface of contact between the upper canine pontic and the lower canine, ensuring that the tooth is intruded vertically.

The lower canine can be intruded using orthodontic movement. This has an added benefit of allowing some degree of retrievability. If the patient is unable to accommodate to the appliance, the brackets could be removed.

If orthodontics or a Dahl is not feasible, occlusal adjustment and reduction of the clinical crown height of the lower canine may produce space for a bridge. If dentine is exposed, a crown might be needed on the lower canine.

● The lateral incisor has a short clinical crown

The lateral incisor is mesially inclined and has a short clinical crown, complicating the bridge design. There is insufficient crown height available for a conventional crown on the lateral incisor and so it is unlikely to produce sufficient retention for a bridge.

Replacement of a canine

The canine is the most technically demanding tooth to replace. The canine has been described as the corner-stone of the mouth. It usually has the longest root and makes an ideal abutment tooth. Correspondingly, the relatively small size of first premolars and lateral incisors usually make these teeth poor abutments.

What are your options for treatment?

Conventional bridge using the premolar and the lateral incisor as abutments.
Simple cantilever bridge using the premolar.
Simple cantilever bridge using both premolars as abutments.
Single tooth implant.
Minimal preparation bridges.

A diagnostic wax-up is needed to provide the dentist and the patient with an indication of the planned definitive restorations. Mounted diagnostic casts give the clinician and the technician an idea of how much space is available on the lingual side.

Conventional bridge using the premolar and the lateral incisor as abutments

The benefit of using retainers on both teeth is that the relative width of the crowns and pontic can be changed to hide the relatively large horizontal space. A diagnostic set-up can be made to assess how much the widths of the abutments and pontics can be altered to provide the optimum appearance for the bridge. If there is some doubt, up to three set-ups can be made to provide the patient with sufficient choice to make an informed decision.

In the present case, the lateral incisor is mesially inclined and has a small crown, making it unsuitable for an abutment. A 2-mm occlusal reduction on the lateral incisor for a crown would leave insufficient tooth for retention of a bridge.

Simple cantilever bridge using the premolar

The premolar is too small and the edentulous space too wide to make this a suitable choice.

Simple cantilever bridge using both premolars as abutments

The premolar is not large enough to support a simple cantilever bridge and the lateral incisor has an unfavourable size. Another choice would be to use both premolars as double abutments. Double abutments reportedly have a higher chance of failure because caries can develop beneath the most distal retainer. Provided care is taken in the design of a double abutment bridge, this can be successful but is usually better avoided. If the teeth have wide and long contact points, the retainers become too close to allow interdental cleaning.

Single tooth implant

An implant would restore the space but the crown will be too wide. The adjacent teeth would need veneers or even crowns to increase their width and so hide the space discrepancy. If the size and shape of the adjacent teeth were accepted, a crown of normal width could be made for the canine, leaving a small diastema distally to hide imbalance in the horizontal space. This would probably be the ideal solution.

Minimal preparation bridges

It is unlikely that minimum preparation bridges would be viable in this case as the premolars have extensive restorations and the lateral incisor is too small.

A conventional crown could be placed on the premolar and a minimum preparation bridge from the palatal surface of the lateral might succeed, but this does not overcome the disparity in the size of the edentulous space.

Generally, distal cantilever bridges should be avoided. The closer a tooth is to the mandibular hinge axis, the greater is the force applied to the occlusal surface, increasing the risk of de-cementation or fracture.

Learning outcomes
- Assessing teeth for bridges.
- Problems with vertical space.
- Replacement of canines.
- Creation of vertical space for restorations.

11

Wide edentulous spaces

Clinical details

This 35-year-old woman requests a bridge to restore the edentulous space in her upper jaw (Fig. 11.1). She has worn a denture for some years and would like a more permanent replacement. There is no dentinal sensitivity.

Clinical observations

- The space between the upper central incisor and the premolar is 12 mm. The edentulous space is wider than a single tooth but narrower than the missing lateral incisor and canine.
- There is tooth wear, mainly erosion, on the palatal surfaces of the upper incisors. The other teeth are unaffected.
- The lip line is favourable.
- There is no evidence of caries or periodontal disease.

What are the complicating factors and how could you manage this case?

Aetiology of the tooth wear.

Horizontal space.

● Aetiology of the tooth wear

The first stage is to identify the cause of the erosion. The two main possibilities are regurgitation of gastric juice or acidic foods and drinks. A dietary history should include

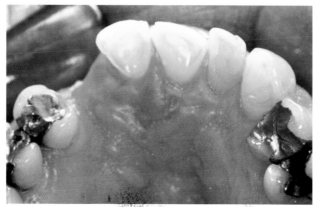

Fig. 11.1 A palatal view of the patient in Case 11.

an analysis of the frequency of consumption of acidic drinks and foods and the presence of any drinking habits that might exacerbate the erosion. Some people drink by holding or swilling acidic liquids in the palatal vault prior to swallowing; others may consume small amounts over very long periods of time. For instance, eating an orange a day may not seem particularly erosive, but it might if the patient ate each piece over 3–4 hours when the potential for erosion would be high.

If a dietary history reveals no obvious cause, other possibilities of tooth wear such as an eating disorder, chronic alcoholism or regurgitation should be investigated. If the aetiology remains undiagnosed, the erosion may continue and further damage may undermine the appearance of the future restorations.

● Horizontal space

The options for the design of restoration are similar to those of Case 10, the major difference being that, in this present case, two teeth are missing rather than one. A choice therefore needs to be made whether to use one or two pontics. Ideally, the appearance should match the contralateral side to ensure that symmetry is maintained, but this is not always feasible. A diagnostic wax-up is essential. If the patient is wearing a partial denture and is content with its appearance, the shape can be copied in the final restoration, even if this means that the edentulous side has two teeth and the opposite side has one.

The first decision should be whether the tooth wear needs treating. If the tooth wear is inactive, the eroded surfaces can be left unrestored and the missing teeth replaced. The only reliable method to determine if the tooth wear is active is to take study models and review the progress of the wear. If the activity cannot be controlled, the dentist must decide at what stage treatment is indicated. Treatment should be considered if the appearance of the teeth are compromised, there is intractable sensitivity, loss of the incisal edge, the tooth wear cannot be controlled and is likely to compromise the remaining tooth structure and, most importantly, the patient's wishes.

In this present case, the degree of tooth wear is not severe. Even though dentine is exposed, it is unlikely that the appearance is compromised and the most important factor to consider is the patient's wishes. The age of the patient is an important consideration. If restorations are placed they are unlikely to last a lifetime and therefore a conservative approach is important. The most conservative treatment is to monitor the wear and prevent further damage.

If the patient accepts restorations, direct composite veneers can be bonded onto the palatal surfaces of the upper incisors. The composites can help to protect the tooth from further erosion. Alternatively, metal onlays made of precious or non-precious alloys cemented onto the palatal surface will provide similar protection, but they may darken the teeth.

What are the options for treatment?

Orthodontics.
Bridges.
Implants.

● Orthodontics

Ideally, the crown replacing the canine and incisor should be the same size as the contralateral side, but this is not possible with the space available. Therefore orthodontics could be used to move teeth and create the ideal widths. Both central incisors are somewhat retroclined, producing a class II division 2 incisal relationship. Fixed orthodontics in the upper and lower jaws might correct the incisal relationship, producing sufficient space for two normally sized teeth. The replacements could be either implants or bridges but symmetry would be conserved.

● Bridges

A conventional fixed-fixed bridge using the incisor and the premolar as abutments to restore the gap

The width of the retainers and pontics could be altered to hide the asymmetry. The edentulous space could be restored with one or two pontics. If one pontic is used, the width of the retainers would be increased. With two pontics, the retainers would be narrower; this is probably the preferred option. First premolars are not ideal retainers; using a double abutment and extending the bridge onto the second premolar is overly destructive.

Two separate, conventional simple cantilever bridges using the central incisor and the premolar

The central incisor would support a distal cantilever bridge while the premolar supported a canine. Since both abutment teeth would be prepared for crowns, there would be flexibility in the width of the teeth, similar to a fixed-fixed bridge design. Using the first premolar as a retainer for a single cantilever bridge is not ideal. Therefore this design is probably not recommended.

Conventional simple cantilever design with double abutments on both premolars

This option would improve the retention for the pontic, but an addition of composite would still be needed on the distal surface of the incisor; this maintains the problem of symmetry and balancing the sizes of the anterior segment and is therefore not an option.

Conventional simple cantilever using the premolar as a retainer

The pontic could replace a normally sized canine, together with a small addition of composite to the distal surface of the upper central incisor.

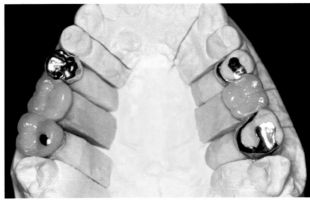

Fig. 11.2 A conventionally designed fixed-fixed bridge on the patient's right side; on the left, a minimally prepared fixed-fixed bridge.

● Implants

This might be sufficient to ensure that the relative sizes of the teeth are balanced. However, the edentulous space is too wide for one implant and too small for two to make this a feasible design. The greatest problem is relying on the premolar to support a normally sized canine, making this option unreliable.

A single tooth implant would be the most conservative of tooth tissue but the replacement crown would still be too wide. Small composite restorations could be added to the mesial and distal surfaces of the adjacent teeth to close the gap. Considering the expense of the implant and the possibility that the composites would stain, it would not be an option. Alternatively, the adjacent teeth could be crowned before the implants are placed and slightly widened, and a slightly wider canine placed in the edentulous space.

How can you classify bridges and what designs are possible?

Bridges can be classified according to the way the teeth are prepared: conventional and minimal preparation. The designs are common to both:

Fixed-fixed (Fig. 11.2).
Fixed-movable (Figs 11.3 and 11.4).

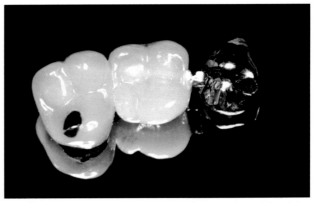

Fig. 11.3 A fixed-movable bridge with a semi-precision joint between the premolar and the molar.

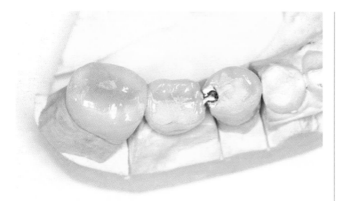

Fig. 11.4 The advantage of a fixed-movable design is that both retainers do not need to be parallel; this overcomes the problem of using teeth with different inclinations.

Cantilever (Fig. 11.5).
Spring cantilever (Fig. 11.6).

● Fixed-fixed

The teeth either side of the edentulous space are directly linked to each other by a rigid connector. The abutment teeth either side of the edentulous space need to have near parallel, but not undercut, surfaces. For a conventional bridge, the tooth preparations should not be undercut on any surface.

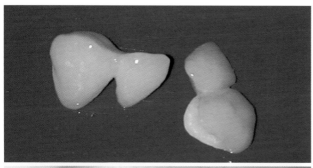

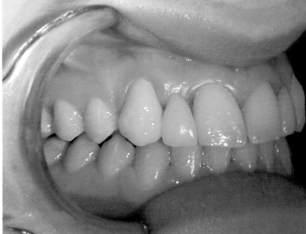

Fig. 11.5 A simple cantilever bridge uses one tooth for support. The canine in this case supports a simple cantilever all-ceramic bridge replacing the lateral incisor.

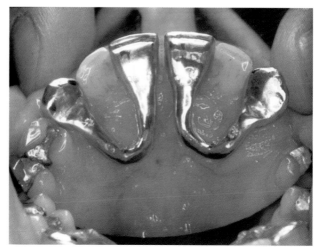

Fig. 11.6 These two spring cantilever bridges using the canines as abutment are an example of an unusual design in that the first molars are more commonly used. More commonly, implants are used to restore the missing teeth and are especially indicated when a mid-line diastema is present.

● Fixed-movable

This is similar to the fixed-fixed design as the abutment teeth are linked, but in this case by a movable joint. The joints can be precision or semi-precision; the former has an improved fit and is rigid whereas the latter allows more flexibility. The major advantage of this type of design over a fixed-fixed design is that the preparations on the abutment teeth need not be parallel to each other (Fig. 11.4). There may be some gain from the slight vertical movement of the joint, which allows the abutment teeth to move independently. Normally, the most distal tooth carries the major retainer but occasionally this is reversed.

● Cantilever

A simple design as the pontic is only supported on one side. Normally, this type of bridge is used to replace single teeth and only one retainer is used to support the bridge. Occasionally, two retainers are used (e.g. in distal cantilever bridges), but the risk of failure is increased, especially from partial de-cementation and caries beneath the retainers.

● Spring cantilever

This is a rarely used design as the pontic is placed some distance away from the retainer. A metal arm links the two parts of the bridge and contacts the hard palate so it is partly supported by soft tissue. Before implants became common, this design was used to replace missing upper anterior teeth with diastemata.

Learning outcomes

- Replacement of canines.
- Managing restorations in patients with tooth wear.
- Classification and design of bridges.

12

Cleft palate

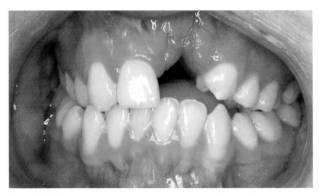

Fig. 12.1 The appearance of the patient in Case 12.

Clinical details

A 24-year-old man presented to your surgery wishing to have his missing anterior teeth replaced with a bridge (Fig. 12.1). There were no medical problems. He had had the cleft palate repaired when he was a child with no further complications. The cleft was restricted to the premaxilla; there was no involvement of the soft palate and the space between the adjacent teeth is 15 mm. He would like to have a fixed replacement for his existing partial denture. What factors should you consider prior to treatment? What special tests might you use to plan the treatment and what are the options? Give reasons for each choice.

Clinical observations

- There is gingival scarring apical to the upper central incisor and the shape of the soft and hard tissue discrepancy supports the history of a cleft.
- There is substantial soft and hard tissue loss in the area of the premaxilla.
- Both lateral incisors and the upper left central incisor and canine are missing.
- The tooth loss is asymmetrical.
- The adjacent teeth are unrestored.
- There is a partial anterior open bite but the upper central incisor is in contact with the opposing teeth.
- There is a bilateral cross bite and a mid-line shift.

What are the potential complicating factors?

Loss of soft and hard tissue.
The lip line.
The length of span of the prosthesis.

Anatomy.
Adjacent teeth.
Occlusion.

● Loss of soft and hard tissue

The patient had a cleft palate repaired when he was a child and this has left a deficiency of soft issue around the edentulous ridge. An advantage of a partial denture is that it replaces soft and hard tissue. The existing partial denture will show the extent of the hard tissue loss by the amount of acrylic used in the buccal flange. A bridge replacing the missing teeth might not improve the appearance. Long pontics would have to be made to hide the missing tissue or the patient would have to accept a gap between the base of the pontic and the gingival tissues if the pontics were kept to a normal length.

● The lip line

The position of the upper lip line is critical for anterior bridges. If a patient has a high lip line (i.e. the cervical margins are visible when smiling), particular care should be taken on placing the margins on the crowns or the location of the pontics. Different types of pontics can be used to hide this appearance but they are not always successful. Patients with cleft lip and palates have scarring around the circumoral tissues, resulting in a tight lip and consequently a low lip line, which often hides the margins of the crowns.

● The length of span of the prosthesis

In this case, the length of span is shorter than the width of three normally sized teeth (see Table 12.1). In a person without a cleft, orthodontics could be used to create a symmetrical appearance, possibly by retracting the posterior teeth, correcting any mid-line shift and

Table 12.1 Average width of teeth (mm)

	Central incisor	Lateral incisor	Canine	First premolar	Second premolar	First molar	Second molar
Maxilla	8.5	6.5	8	7	6.5	10	9.5
Mandible	5.5	6	7	7	7	11	10.5

creating sufficient space for replacement teeth of ideal width. In this case, orthodontics will not be possible because of the absence of alveolar bone in the edentulous premaxilla.

● Anatomy

The loss of alveolar bone in the premaxilla is one complicating factor, but so too is the position of the incisive canal. Normally, this is palatal to and mid-way between the upper central incisors. A large incisive canal can prevent the use of implants as there is insufficient bone to allow osseo-integration.

● Adjacent teeth

Both potential abutment teeth are unrestored and are not tilted or rotated. However, the presence of the upper premolar in the canine position increases the demand on the clinician to create the optimum appearance.

● Occlusion

The bilateral cross bite is consistent with a cleft palate caused by a hypoplastic maxilla. Corrective surgery in the first few years of life can hinder normal growth through scar formation, producing a hypoplastic maxilla. The open bite is between the left premolars and the lower arch, whilst the right central incisor has an occlusal contact.

What special tests might you choose?

Radiographic examination.
Study models and diagnostic wax-ups.

● Radiographic examination

This depends to some extent on what treatment is envisaged. Periapical radiographs are needed of the potential abutment teeth and edentulous space. The incisive canal should be identified and its size and position compared to any potential implant fixture sites. Most implant manufacturers provide transparent real-sized line drawings of different sized fixtures that can be superimposed onto a radiograph to determine the vertical height of bone.

● Study models and diagnostic wax-ups

Considering the occlusal relationship, it is questionable whether articulated study casts are necessary as the presence of the anterior open bite reduces the complexity of any prosthesis, but casts mounted on a semi-adjustable articulator may aid the treatment planning. Although the anterior guidance will be predominantly on the cusps of the molars and right premolars, the tips of the incisors may make some contribution, especially towards the end of the movement. An existing partial denture will provide the ideal diagnostic aid provided it fulfils the demands of the patient. Waxing-up teeth on the study models is another method used to assess the ideal number of pontics needed to bridge the edentulous space.

In this case, it is likely that two pontics will be possible and therefore the decision needs to be taken as to which teeth would provide the best appearance. The choices are a central incisor and a canine or a central and lateral incisor; often the former option is more successful, especially so in this case as the contralateral lateral incisor is also missing.

What are the options for treatment?

Bridges
- A fixed-fixed bridge from incisor to premolar.
- A cantilever bridge using the premolar or the incisor as the abutment, with recontouring of the adjacent teeth.

Implants
- Single-tooth implant with recontouring of the premolar and incisor.
- Two implants replacing two teeth in the edentulous area with or without reshaping or stripping of the proximal surfaces of the adjacent teeth.

Denture
- Two teeth replaced with a cobalt–chrome framework or an acrylic resin base.
- Three teeth replaced with a cobalt–chrome framework or an acrylic resin base.

● Bridges

A conventional or minimally prepared bridge could be used to restore the edentulous space. A minimally prepared simple cantilever bridge would be relatively simple to prepare on the premolar because there is no contact with the opposing teeth, but the situation is more complex on the central incisor as the teeth are in contact. To avoid the pontic being too wide, some improvement to the appearance may be possible by placing a veneer or composite addition onto the distal surface of the incisor.

A conventional bridge, either a fixed-fixed design or simple cantilever, would need preparations on the premolar and/or the incisor; this could be considered a disadvantage as both teeth are unrestored. A simple cantilever conventional bridge would have no advantage over a minimal preparation bridge. The fixed-fixed design would involve crown preparations on both the incisor and the premolar and therefore the relative widths of the retainers and the pontic could be changed to provide optimum aesthetics. This might not overcome the problem of asymmetry caused by the width of the edentulous space.

Alternatively, two narrower teeth, for a conventional fixed-fixed bridge, could be placed in the edentulous space; this would eliminate the need for reshaping the premolar or incisor but it too produces asymmetry.

● Implants

The major difficulty with implants is the relative absence of alveolar bone in the cleft site. A single-tooth implant in

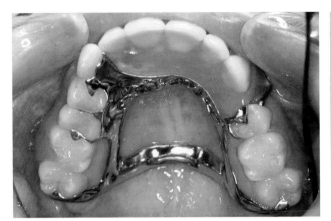

Fig. 12.2 A Kennedy class IV partial denture.

the central incisor position would not overcome the demands of the width of the space. Addition of composite/porcelain veneers onto the adjacent teeth might hide the asymmetry, but the overall appearance of the restorations would rely on the composite bond. The weakest link in the restoration of the space would be the composite or porcelain margin and once this had stained the restoration would become unacceptable. Two

implants, one in the central incisor position and the other in the lateral/canine position, would replace two teeth, but the amount of space is critical (see Box 21.1).

Partial dentures

If the patient has a low lip line, any restoration without soft tissue replacement may be unacceptable. Kennedy class IV dentures replacing anterior teeth are one of the more clinically demanding types of denture. An example of a design is shown in Fig. 12.2. The appearance of the acrylic to tooth junction on the mesial aspect of the central incisor is critical to avoid the formation of a dark triangle of space. The denture may need an angled path of insertion to optimize the appearance of the flange of the denture.

Learning outcomes

- Planning anterior restorations involving alveolar bone loss.
- Using special tests.
- Replacing single missing anterior teeth.
- Average width of teeth.

13

Replacing posterior teeth

Clinical details

The upper first molar became grade III mobile and the patient lost the tooth 6 months ago. He was diagnosed as having rapidly progressive periodontal disease, which is now treated and is under control. There was no complicating medical history, but the patient smokes 20 cigarettes a day. The patient would like to have the tooth replaced but is not prepared to fund the cost of implants (Fig. 13.1). What is your management?

Clinical observations

- There is a moderately extensive restoration in the second molar, whereas the premolar is unrestored; both teeth are caries-free.
- The edentulous space is one molar unit wide.
- The occlusal surfaces of the molar are not involved in guidance.
- There is sufficient width and height of bone for an implant.

What are the potential complicating factors?

Extraction site.
Smoking.
Finance.

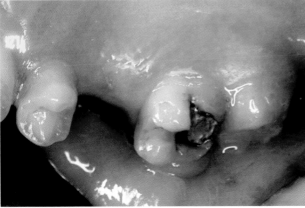

Fig. 13.1 The appearance of the edentulous space in Case 13.

● Extraction site

The patient had the tooth extracted 6 months previously, which would be considered sufficient time for alveolar bony remodelling to occur. Although there is a risk that further alveolar bone resorption may occur and that a gap develops beneath the pontic, the chances are less considering the time since the extraction.

● Smoking

It is recognized that smoking increases the risk of failure of the osseo-integration of implant fixtures. Nicotine and other products inhaled in cigarette smoke increase the chance of failure by a factor of about two. Nicotine causes vasoconstriction in peripheral vessels and consequently reduces peripheral circulation in the gingival tissues. In patients with chronic periodontal disease, this results in reduced bleeding on probing and may lead to a clinical impression that the disease is less advanced. Some authorities recommend advising patients to stop smoking 2–3 weeks prior to surgery, but such is the compulsive nature of the habit that this may not be achieved. Patients who smoke and are considering implants must accept the increased risk and so clinicians should record these details carefully in the notes.

● Finance

The patient is unable to fund the cost of implants. The patient should be informed about implants, even if he cannot afford them. The lifetime costs of implants are probably cheaper than replacing bridges. Some insurance schemes may consider funding implants.

Special tests

The only special tests needed would be periapical radiographs and vitality tests of the abutment teeth. The electric pulp test is considered the most reliable of all the vitality tests. This involves passing electrical stimuli through the tooth, a positive result indicating that a nerve supply is present.

What are the options for treatment?

A bridge is the only treatment possible given the patient's preferences (Fig. 13.2). Either a conventionally prepared bridge or a minimally prepared bridge could replace the missing tooth. A conventional, full-coverage crown preparation on the unrestored second premolar is considered overly destructive. A conventional retainer could be made for the molar with a minimally prepared, resin-bonded retainer on the premolar. However, in this case, a minimally prepared bridge using a fixed-movable design was used to replace the missing tooth.

The maximum surface area has been used for bonding. Part of the existing amalgam restoration was removed and the surfaces rendered caries-free and then extended onto the distal surface. The preparation could be described as a hybrid bridge. The movable joint allows some movement of the abutment teeth and also eliminates the need for parallel preparations. The metal is about 1 mm thick and is placed onto sound tooth surface, cemented and then adjusted to ensure a comfortable fit. The joint is precision-cast and allows a vertical path of insertion. The disadvantage of this type of bridge is that the metal surface may be visible when smiling. This problem, however, is less likely in the maxilla. Another possibility is that the retainer on the premolar may debond. The pontic has a saddle-shaped design.

What are the design principles of minimal preparation bridges?

Normally, minimal preparation bridges are used to replace single teeth. The bridges gain their retention from the bond between the metal and the tooth surface. Early types of luting cements had no or little dentine-bonding capability, but the more recent improved types give bond strengths to dentine that are similar to those to enamel.

● Preparation

Lack of occlusal space

If the opposing teeth are in contact, space is needed for the retainer. This can be created either by removing tooth tissue or by cementing the retainer high. Preparations may expose vital dentine, but the bond strengths of modern adhesives to dentine are sufficiently reliable to retain the bridge. If the retainer is cemented high, forcing intrusion/extrusion of teeth to create the space normally takes a few weeks.

Insufficient surface area

Small teeth may have insufficient surface area for bonding. Additional surface area can be gained by preparing rest seats or grooves/slots. This also increases the rigidity of

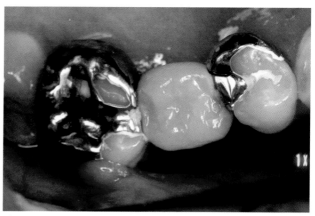

Fig. 13.2 A minimally prepared bridge using a fixed-movable design with partial coverage retainers on both abutment teeth and a saddle-shaped pontic.

the bridge, which is even more important for a successful restoration. The location of slots/grooves or rest seats can also aid accurate positioning during cementation.

Restored abutment teeth

Provided the restorations are minimal, they can be removed and incorporated into the design of the bridge (Fig. 13.2). Additionally, using existing cavities means that the rigidity of the bridge is increased. In some instances, the design may approach that of a conventional bridge but less tooth tissue is removed. Recent research suggests that, for minimal preparation bridges, preparing the teeth improves their longevity.

● Occlusal design

For most bridges, a conformative approach is chosen as the most convenient occlusal scheme. The canines guide the mandible in lateral excursions and produce posterior disclusion (Box 13.1). This makes the design of the occlusal table of the pontics simpler. When group function is

---

Box 13.1 Designing the occlusion for complex crown and bridge

When designing the occlusal scheme for multiple crowns or bridges, the most convenient is canine-guided, creating posterior disclusion on lateral excursions. Anterior guidance should be shared on the palatal surfaces of the upper incisors, producing posterior disclusion. This occlusal scheme is usually selected because it is easier to make in the laboratory. Creating group function to guide lateral excursions is more demanding on the technician since the occlusal form of the posterior teeth has to be relatively flat and each guiding surface needs to be carefully formed so that interferences do not hinder the free movement of the mandible in lateral excursions. For this reason, canine guidance is normally used when re-organizing occlusion.

For a conformative occlusal scheme, crowns should not interfere or produce early points of contact by other teeth or crowns. The occlusion remains in the intercuspal position. For a re-organized approach, the contact of teeth to crowns or crowns to crowns should be evenly distributed.

Occlusal contacts should therefore be even in distribution and spread over as many teeth or crowns as possible. Anterior guidance should be taken by the palatal surfaces of the incisors and lateral excursions should be guided by the palatal surface of canines.

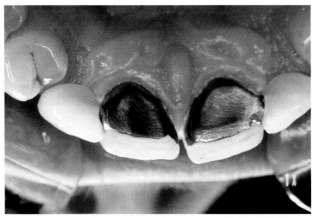

Fig. 13.3 The retainers cover the maximum surface area available for bonding on the central incisors. The retainer passes around the medial mesial edge, not so far as to become visible but sufficient to increase the rigidity of the framework. Often these bridges fail because the metal flexes under strain and debonds. The more rigid the framework, the less this is likely to occur. The pontic is a ridge lap design which allows easy cleaning but does not restore the tooth shape.

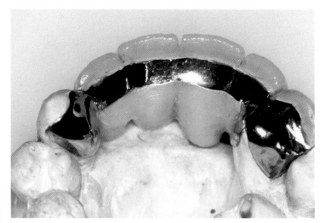

Fig. 13.4 A modified ridge lap design conserves the lingual shape of teeth and yet provides sufficient space for cleaning beneath the pontics.

involved in lateral excursions, the occlusal design is more difficult as it must conform. Therefore the design of the occlusal surface of a pontic or retainer is more complex.

● Cementation

The most difficult stage in placing minimally prepared bridges is their cementation. If the teeth have been prepared with slots/grooves or rest seats, these will help to seat the bridge during cementation. Occlusal adjustment can be difficult to accomplish before cementation and is most successfully achieved after. A dry working field is necessary for adhesive cements. This can often be achieved with judicious use of cotton wool rolls but, if adequate moisture control cannot be obtained, a rubber dam will help.

What are the preferred designs for anterior and posterior bridges?

Anterior bridges (Fig. 13.3).
Posterior bridges (Fig. 13.4).

● Anterior bridges

The design of choice to replace upper anterior teeth is the simple cantilever. An exception may follow orthodontic treatment, where a fixed-fixed design is recommended to provide a splinting action. Fixed-fixed designs are preferred for replacing lower incisors.

● Posterior bridges

Any design can be used, but the most successful is the fixed-movable. This eliminates the need for parallel surfaces either side of the edentulous space whilst allowing some independent movement of the abutment teeth, a factor that significantly reduces the risk of retainer de-cementation.

What are the types of pontic design?

Ridge lap.
Modified ridge lap.
Dome-shaped.
Saddle-shaped.
Ovate.
Wash-through.

● Ridge lap

The shape of the buccal surface matches the adjacent teeth but the lingual surface is cut away to allow access for cleaning. Whilst the appearance is maintained, the patient may complain that only half the tooth has been replaced. If a patient is susceptible to periodontal disease, this is a safer option (Fig. 13.3).

● Modified ridge lap

This is a compromise on a ridge lap, with more of the lingual shape being preserved but still allowing the patient to clean under the pontic, and may be better tolerated (Fig. 13.4).

● Dome-shaped or bullet-shaped

Dome- or bullet-shaped pontics have a point contact with the edentulous ridge. This design can be particularly useful when the apical third of the pontic is not visible (e.g. in lower premolars).

● Saddle-shaped

This a more realistic tooth shape, with a concave surface on the gingival surface. The U-shaped surface increases the difficulty of cleaning but, for patients with excellent oral hygiene and who are resistant to periodontal disease, it may prove the most acceptable design (Fig. 13.5).

● Ovate

This is a similar shape to the saddle shape but is designed to place pressure on the edentulous ridge to change the shape of the ridge. It may be used as part of a provisional

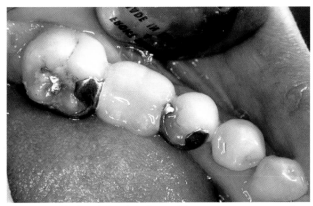

Fig. 13.5 This fixed-fixed design utilizes rest seat preparations on the abutment teeth to increase the surface for bonding as well as the rigidity of the retainer. The disadvantage of this design is that the surfaces adjacent to the pontic need to be virtually parallel in order to avoid undercuts preventing location of the bridge.

bridge to scallop and contour the edentulous ridges prior to placement of the definitive restoration.

● Wash-through

Here, there is no contact between the pontic and the ridge. This type of pontic is not commonly used as the

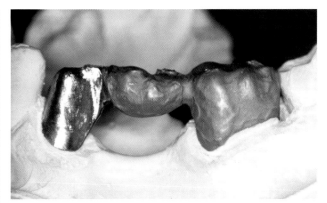

Fig. 13.6 A sanitary pontic or wash-through does not replace the appearance of a missing tooth but does help restore function.

shape of the tooth is not replicated, merely its occlusal form (Fig. 13.6). Other terms used for this type of pontic are hygienic or sanitary pontics.

Learning outcomes

- Management of single missing posterior teeth.
- Designing minimal preparation bridges.
- Pontic design.
- Occlusal design.

14

Replacing upper incisors

Clinical details

This 35-year-old man presents to your surgery requesting an alternative to his acrylic resin partial denture which replaces four maxillary incisors (Fig. 14.1). He lost these teeth as a result of trauma when he was a teenager and has worn a partial denture ever since. The current denture is over 5 years old, has broken once and has become loose. Despite these shortcomings, the patient copes quite well with the prosthesis. He is a non-smoker and has a clear medical history. He has an otherwise unrestored dentition and there is no evidence of caries.

Clinical observations

- The periodontal condition and remaining dentition is healthy.
- The standard of oral hygiene is fair. Gingival bleeding upon probing is evident around the denture abutment teeth.
- The maxillary canine teeth are vital, unrestored and their long axes are parallel to each other.
- The edentulous alveolar ridge between the maxillary canines is well formed, having undergone minimal resorption.
- There is an optimum lip line and the gingival tissues do not show on smiling.

What options are available to effectively restore the edentulous space and what problems are associated with each choice?

Implants.
Conventional bridge.
Partial denture.

● Implants

In this situation the prospects for successful treatment with implants are good. There has been minimal alveolar ridge resorption between the maxillary canines and the patient is not a smoker. Further investigations, including 3D radiographic imaging, would be necessary to confirm adequate bone volume and quality.

The placement of implants in the incisor position can be complicated by the presence of the incisive foramen. This is particularly so if the foramen is large and buccally placed. In such situations, it is usually more convenient to place two fixtures in the lateral incisor position and use them as retainers for a fixed-fixed bridge to replace the two central incisors. An alternative approach would be to place four single tooth implants, provided the bone support is adequate, the incisive canal is conveniently situated and it does not interfere with the symmetry.

● Conventional bridge

The edentulous space is too wide for minimal preparation bridges and therefore the only option is conventional bridgework. A conventional, metal–ceramic bridge would be an acceptable restoration. It would normally involve full coverage crown retainers on the canines only. Some clinicians consider it necessary to recruit the first premolars into the design, but this is a minority view. The major complication of this type of prosthesis is the extent of the tooth reduction necessary to accommodate the crown retainers. There is a risk of pulpal damage and necrosis over the short or long term. The alternative approach of using a resin-bonded bridge would be considered by

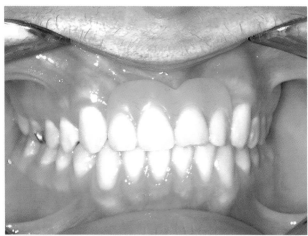

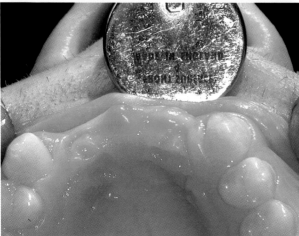

Fig. 14.1 Case 14 with and without the denture. It is important to feel the width of the buccal edentulous ridge. Extraction of the incisors can lead to significant bone loss, resulting in insufficient bone in the area where implants are planned.

many clinicians to be extending this technology beyond its limits. However, a combination of evolving design concepts and improving cements has, in selected cases, made long-span resin-bonded bridgework a realistic possibility. The long-term performance of resin-bonded bridges can be maximized by incorporating, where possible, the following design features:

Maximum coverage by the retaining wings of the abutment teeth.
Supplementary slots and grooves.
Making the casting as rigid as possible.

Clinical experience with resin-bonded bridgework has shown that cantilever designs are, for the most part, very successful. In this case, however, a fixed-fixed construction is required in order to resist torsional forces.

● Partial dentures

Acrylic resin partial denture

The most common design of acrylic resin partial denture involves the intimate contact of the denture base with the palatal dentogingival junctions of many, if not all, of the remaining teeth in the same arch. Increased plaque accumulation, food impaction and sometimes direct trauma contribute to increased levels of gingival inflammation and hyperplasia. In the absence of effective oral hygiene, caries and periodontal disease can be significantly accelerated. For these reasons, this design of partial denture is best avoided.

In certain situations, acrylic resin partial dentures can be designed in such a way as to avoid the majority of the dentogingival junctions and so reduce the risk of compromising the health of the remaining teeth. An example is the Every denture, which, although originally designed to replace single maxillary incisors, can sometimes be modified to include more replacement teeth.

The present case would be suitable for such a prosthesis as the buccal segment teeth are intact, space is available for ball-ended clasps to engage the distal surfaces of the last standing upper molars, there is space for a labial flange and the palate is relatively shallow.

Metal-based partial denture

Metal-based partial dentures are usually made from a combination of cobalt–chromium alloy and heat-cured acrylic resin. Successful design of a Kennedy class IV prosthesis (see Fig. 12.2) requires careful attention to the path of insertion of the denture and the placement of components that provide tooth support and direct and indirect retention. A well-designed and accurately constructed skeleton framework metal partial denture can be a very successful means of replacing missing anterior teeth.

Metal-based partial dentures with precision attachments

Precision attachments would improve the retention of the partial denture, probably avoiding the use of anterior

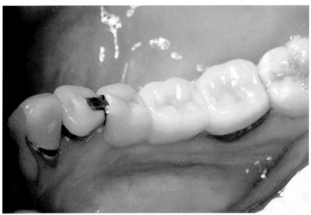

Fig. 14.2 A fixed-movable bridge from the second molar to the first premolar. In this case, the attachment is precision-made to allow a rigid connector between the two components.

clasps. However, they are bulky and need a relatively long clinical crown to support their length, although shorter attachments are available.

What are precision attachments?

The most common form of retention for dentures is usually clasps. However, if the shape of the crowns contain little or no undercut, clasping teeth to gain retention can be unsuitable. Clasps also have the disadvantage that they are generally visible. Precision attachments are either intra- or extracoronal and provide retention from the close fit between the male and female parts and along the path of withdrawal (Fig. 14.2). Semi-precision attachments provide less retention but reduce the stress upon the teeth (see Fig. 11.4). The most common design of precision attachment is the ball and socket (Fig. 14.3). Precision attachments have found increased use with implant-retained dentures.

What is the role of a provisional restoration and how might you make one?

A provisional bridge has a number of functions. It will assess the success of:

The bridge design over the short to medium term.
The position of the incisal edge relative to the lips.
The shape and, if possible, colour of the pontics.
The anterior guidance and lateral excursions.
The emergence shape of the abutment teeth.

The simplest temporary restoration would be individual crowns on the canines and to leave the edentulous space unrestored, but this will not assess success of the bridge design. A provisional bridge can be made by taking an impression of the diagnostic wax-up with a silicone material to produce a matrix, which can then be relocated into the patient's mouth after tooth preparations and loaded with a temporary bridge material. Another method is to copy the diagnostic wax-up in dental stone and make a vacuum-formed splint over the model. This transparent rigid material is placed over the tooth

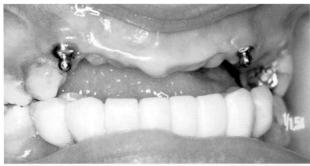
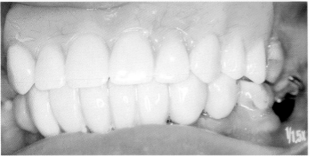

Fig. 14.3 A two-ball and socket precision attachment placed in the canine position helps to retain the partial denture.

preparations. The flow of the provisional bridge material is more easily assessed and reduces the potential for air-blows, which can occur with non-transparent matrices. Provisional crowns or bridges are usually made from composite, but can also be made in acrylic.

What are the stages in fitting crowns or bridges?

Fit surface.
Margins.
Contact points.
Occlusion.
Appearance.

● The fit surface

During the casting process, minute blow holes may be formed. If the surfaces are raised, they can potentially interfere with the close fitting of the crown or bridge and need to be removed. Fine dry powder sprayed onto the fitting surface should highlight them.

● Margins of the crown

During the casting process, excess metal or porcelain may be left along the margin. If these remain, they can interfere with the fit of the crown on the tooth.

● Contact points

Although the contact points will probably be adjusted on the model, it is not unusual to find that the crown cannot be seated in the mouth. This is often due to slight abrasion of the stone model or movement of the die while making the crown. Adjustment of the crown can be made by highlighting the areas of early contact with carefully placed articulating paper or dry powder and removing these areas; the surface can then be polished.

● Occlusion

Once fitted, the occlusion of the opposing teeth on the crown or bridge should be checked. Occasionally, this is found to be accurate and may reflect the careful registration of the occlusion together with use of an articulator in the manufacturing process. More usually, slight adjustments are needed. Thin articulating paper should be inserted between the restoration and the opposing tooth and the patient asked to close in either the RCP (retruded contact position) or ICP (intercuspal position), depending upon the occlusal position to which the restoration has been made. The occlusal surface is adjusted until the restoration does not interfere with either the ICP or lateral guidance.

● Appearance

Normally for gold crowns the appearance is not a major part of the assessment, but this is not true for tooth-coloured restorations. A single anterior crown surrounded by natural unrestored teeth is the most difficult crown to match. Ideally, the shade of the restoration should be taken before tooth preparation; this should be in natural light, or with artificial light that has filters to make the light source produce light similar to daylight. Slight alterations in the colour of the crown are possible, usually the addition of surface characteristics or creating lighter shades, but more pronounced changes are difficult to adjust and may need a re-make. If new porcelain is added, the crown will need re-firing.

What are the steps in fitting long-span bridges?

The majority of stages are similar to fitting a crown; the only major difference is ensuring that the occlusion is correct and that the retainers are fully seated on the abutment teeth. If a fixed-movable design is used, the minor retainer, with the female attachment, should be fitted first and thereafter the major retainer. The occlusion should be checked so that both sides of the dentition contact evenly with and without the bridge in place. If the unrestored teeth either side of the bridge are in the same contact positions with and without the bridge, then the bridge is fully adjusted into ICP or RCP, depending on the design of the occlusal scheme. Lateral excursions should be checked to ensure movement occurs without interference from either working or non-working side contacts.

Learning outcomes

- Restoration of an anterior edentulous space.
- Understanding the basics of precision attachments.
- Role of the provision bridge.
- Stages in fitting crowns and bridges.

15

Partial denture design

Clinical history

This 65-year-old patient presents requesting a new lower partial denture to replace an acrylic one, made 10 years ago, which has become loose and unstable. She has an otherwise intact upper dentition (Fig. 15.1). She is currently taking medication to control hypertension and has a history of bleeding postoperatively following extractions. There is no other relevant medical history. What treatment is possible to restore the missing teeth? Describe the principles of designing free-end saddle dentures.

Clinical observations

- She is edentulous distal to the lower premolar.
- The remaining teeth have crowns and extensive amalgams.
- There is a minor amount of tooth wear on her lower incisors.
- She would prefer to have a more stable denture.

What are the options for treatment?

Implant-supported bridge.
Replacement partial dentures.

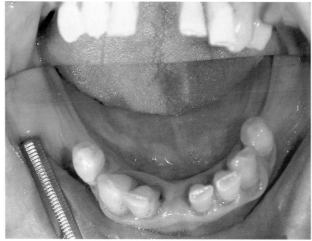

Fig. 15.1 The appearance of the patient in Case 15.

Treatment will depend mostly on what the patient wants, but all the options should be explained, even if she is unlikely to be able to fund implants.

● Implant-supported bridge

Normally, in the mandible there is sufficient bone present for implants. In the maxilla the size of the sinus and the amount of resorption following tooth loss often compromises the placement of implants. If implants were selected as the appropriate restorative treatment, the next stage would be to assess if sufficient bone was present. If the patient has an existing partial denture, metal balls or studs can be temporarily attached to the denture before arranging the radiographs. The metal balls would give an indication of the amount of vertical bone, but they do not provide the same amount of information about the horizontal component. Specialist radiographs, such as CT (computed tomography) scans or Scanora (Nobel Biocare, Sweden), give tomographic sections of the mandible and enable the clinician to assess if sufficient bone exists for implants and their likely relationship to the inferior dental canal.

Considering the number of teeth lost, three implant fixtures would be necessary. Whilst the more mesial implants would approach the optimum length of 10–13 mm, the more distal implant approaching the retromolar region would be unlikely to be above 8 mm. In this case, the patient preferred not to have implants and requested a more-stable partial denture.

● Partial denture

Either a replacement acrylic partial denture or a metal-based one could be offered to the patient. However, another acrylic denture is unlikely to overcome the problem of support and retention; therefore, despite the increased cost, a metal base would provide better comfort for the patient. The patient has a Kennedy Class I denture (see Box 15.1).

What are the stages in designing a partial denture?

Outline the saddle areas.
Place the occlusal rest seats for support.
Place the clasps for direct retention.
Place the indirect retainers.
Connect the denture.

● Occlusal rests

The rest transmits the occlusal load vertically down the long axis of the tooth and aids the support of the denture. Normally, the rests are placed either side of the edentulous space to provide optimum support. If this is not possible, the position is not particularly imperative in the maxilla, but the concept of the RPI (see below and Fig. 15.2) is generally selected in the mandible. The rest seat preparation should have sufficient depth to allow the

Box 15.1 Kennedy classification of partial dentures

Class I: bilateral free-end saddle (Fig. 15.2)

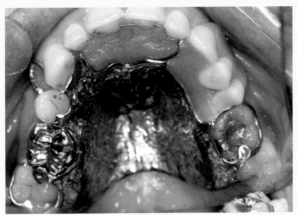

Fig. 15.2 This figure shows a distal extension saddle on the left side. The RPI system (rest, proximal plate, 'I' bar) should provide support and retention without excessive stress on the distal abutment.

Class II: unilateral free-end saddle (Fig. 15.3)

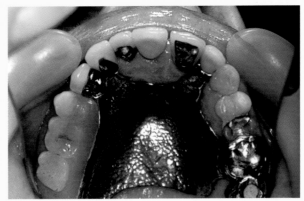

Fig. 15.3 Unilateral free-end saddle, Kennedy class II.

Class III: bounded posterior saddle (Fig. 15.4)

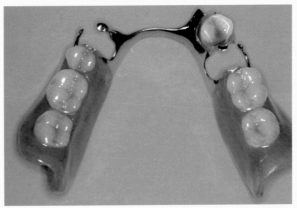

Fig. 15.4 Bounded posterior saddle, Kennedy class III.

Class IV: bounded anterior saddle (Fig. 15.5)

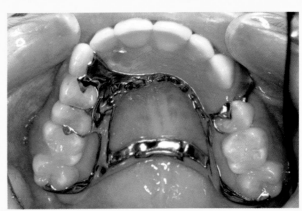

Fig. 15.5 A Kennedy class IV bounded anterior saddle. Note that the rest seats have been placed distally on the last standing molars to increase the indirect retention and so reduce the potential for rotation of the denture.

laboratory technician the necessary space to construct the components. The clinician should assess if adequate space is available while designing the denture. It is neither appropriate nor comfortable for the patient if the initial point of contact on closure is a cast rest. The partial denture should conform to the existing occlusal relationship and be otherwise almost undetectable by the patient. In some situations, the occlusal rest can be an overlay totally enveloping the tooth within the denture. This can provide tremendous support and, if the rest is continued over the buccal and lingual cusps, will contribute to the retention.

● Direct retention

The type of clasp will to some extent depend on the amount of undercut present, which is determined from the casts and the surveying (Fig. 15.6). Although the amount of undercut is not quite as critical as it once was, it is still important. Small composite additions can be bonded onto the labial surfaces to create artificial undercuts for a cobalt–chromium clasp. The clasps resist displacement in a vertical direction.

A long clasp made of any material will be more flexible than a shorter one. If the clasp is too flexible then little retention is gained; conversely, if the clasp is too rigid, it

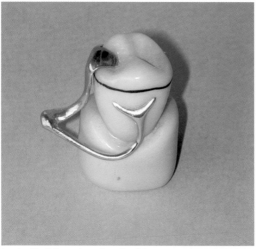 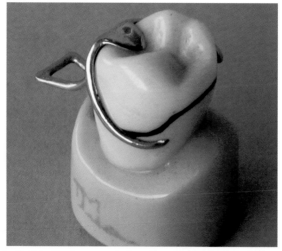

(a) (b)

Fig. 15.6 Gingivally (a) and occlusally (b) approaching clasps. Note that both clasps are below the survey line to ensure sufficient retention. The width of the undercut below the survey line is important and will to some extent determine the material of the clasp. Too large a gap and a cobalt–chromium clasp may not have sufficient flexibility and so may break. The depth of undercut relative to the path of insertion must be less than 0.1 mm for a cobalt–chromium 'I' bar or 0.25 mm for occlusally approaching clasps. Large gaps may require a more flexible material such as a wrought wire.

will be difficult to place in and out. Cobalt–chromium clasps are more rigid than those made from cast or wrought gold; however, gold is more expensive and, although it has certain advantages, the cost often precludes its routine use. The most common clasp designs are occlusally and gingivally approaching clasps. A clasp must also have a bracing arm to allow the force applied to the tooth to be activated; if the clasp is not opposed by another element it will not be activated.

● **Indirect retention**

The displacement from rotational forces is resisted by indirect retention. This is designed into a denture by identifying the major clasp axis and placing an additional rest as far away as practically possible and including a clasp.

● **Connect the denture**

In the present case, the connector will be cobalt–chromium to provide cost-effective rigidity to the denture base. In the mandible, the denture is connected along the lower anterior teeth either by a lingual plate or by a lingual/sublingual bar.

Design of a cobalt partial framework denture

An anterior acrylic flange should extend to the labial sulcus and remain in contact with the buccal mucosa. This will optimize lip support and aesthetics while significantly assisting with the stability of the denture. The shape, size and direction of the labial flange is dictated by the morphology of the edentulous alveolar process which in turn dictates the denture's path of insertion.

Direct retainers are ideally placed on those teeth closest to the edentulous saddle. These may be 'I' bars on the canines or occlusally approaching clasps on the first premolars. Similarly, tooth support for the denture

should be gained from rests extending onto the cingulae of the canines or the mesial marginal ridges of the first premolars. The denture base needs to be extended posteriorly to allow rests to be placed on the occlusal surfaces of the distal teeth in the arch in order to maximize tooth support as well as providing indirect retention.

What is understood by the term RPI?

The RPI (rest, proximal plate, 'I' bar) is a design concept for providing support, retention and the least stress on the distal abutment tooth (Fig. 15.2).

The rest is placed on the mesial aspect of the tooth adjacent to the edentulous saddle. This position, in relation to the 'I' bar clasp, provides a modest degree of indirect retention.

The minor connector between the rest and the lingual bar engages the mesial surface of the abutment tooth and helps resist distal movement of the denture framework.

The 'I' bar provides the direct retention by engaging an undercut in the mid-buccal surface. Being distal to the rest, displacement of the saddle during function results in the clasp being disengaged in a gingival direction, so reducing stress on the tooth.

The proximal plate abuts a guide plane on the distal surface of the abutment tooth to give the denture a single path of insertion and, in conjunction with the mesial rest and minor connector, contributes to the reciprocation of the clasp.

What are the reasons for altering the path of insertion of partial dentures?

Appearance.

Interference.

Retention.

● Appearance

For example, on an anterior saddle, if a partial denture has a vertical path of insertion, an unsightly gap can appear between the saddle and abutment teeth. Giving the cast a posterior tilt, and thus an angled path of insertion, means that the denture flange can extend into the buccal sulcus, so hiding the gap.

● Interference

Using a similar example to the one above, if a hard tissue undercut is present in the premaxillary area, the cast can be tilted to engage the undercut and prevent an interference being present.

● Retention

Often this is confused with tilting a model to create an undercut for a clasp, which is not possible. What can be achieved by tilting a model is the use of proximal tooth surfaces for guide planes.

What impression materials can be used for partial and complete dentures?

Alginates.
Zinc oxide–eugenol.
Impression plaster.
Impression compound.
Mucostatic and mucocompressive (mucodisplacive) impression techniques.

● Alginates

Alginate is the most commonly used type of impression material. It is not dimensionally stable and should be cast shortly after the impression has been taken. Alginates vary considerably in their viscosity. The material is elastic when set and therefore indicated for undercut areas. An impression should record accurately all the necessary anatomy. Care should be taken over the pouring of the model. Areas of impression material that are unsupported should be removed as they can cause distortion of the working model. A special spaced and perforated tray is recommended if alginate is to be used for the secondary impression.

● Zinc oxide–eugenol

This is an accurate impression material which is dimensionally stable but a little messy. The special tray needs to be close-fitting to the primary casts. The impression material is suitable for the edentulous maxilla or mandible but not indicated for undercut areas. It can be used in partially dentate cases when taking an altered cast impression.

● Impression plaster

This material is rarely used these days for the edentulous maxilla. It is capable of producing a very accurate impression, but in areas of undercut will, on removal of the

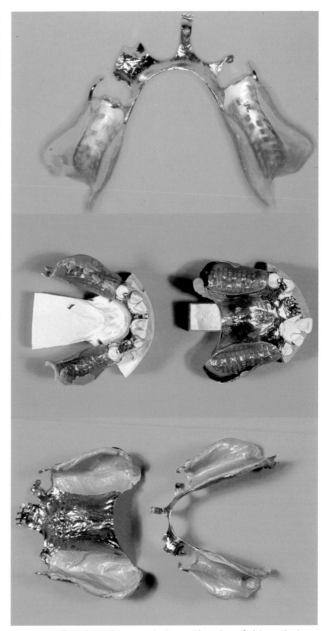

Fig. 15.7 The altered cast technique. The aim of this technique is to overcome the difference between the hard support given by teeth and the more resilient support given by the soft tissues. The conventional impression technique is used to make the metal framework. Over the distal extensions a special tray is added, onto which a viscostatic impression is taken. The operator holds the metal-work over the hard tissues and allows a viscostatic impression of the soft tissue using the special tray. There is some doubt over the usefulness of this technique in view of modern impression techniques.

impression, break off and require re-attachment. It is not suitable for a lower impression as the patient's saliva mixes with the plaster, producing a rough and friable surface.

● Impression compound

This thermoplastic material softens between 55°C and 70°C. Its high viscosity and rigid nature make it an ideal material for extending the periphery of stock trays. A variation in the technique for the edentulous maxilla is to take the impression in two stages: first with impression compound and then alginate over the impression to perfect the surface detail.

● Mucostatic and mucocompressive (mucodisplacive) impression techniques

The ideal impression material should accurately record the surface detail of the mucosa and other related structures. The mucosa overlying the palate is not uniform in thickness and therefore, theoretically, this may affect the accuracy of the impression. A mucostatic impression will record the tissues in an undisplaced position, whereas a mucocompressive impression records it under load. Whether any particular impression material can produce either a mucostatic or a mucocompressive technique is debatable and the terms probably have more theoretical status than practical importance.

What is the altered cast technique?

This technique is designed to improve the support of distal extension saddle dentures (Fig. 15.7). It works by placing the denture-bearing tissues of the distal extension saddle under light compression. The added support this achieves reduces the effect of the denture pivoting around the distal rest.

A close-fitting impression tray covering the distal saddle area is attached to the cobalt–chromium casting. After checking and, if necessary, adjusting the periphery of the tray, an impression is taken using a mucodisplacing impression material. A very low viscosity wax was originally described as the impression material but zinc oxide–eugenol if more commonly used for this technique.

The distal extension saddle area of the working model is cut away. The cobalt–chromium casting is fitted back onto the model and a new cast is poured into the distal extension impression tray, hence the name: the altered cast technique.

Learning outcomes

- ● Options to restore the edentulous mandible.
- ● Stages in designing partial dentures.
- ● The meaning of RPI in the design of partial dentures.
- ● Reasons for altering the path of insertion of dentures.
- ● Impressions used for partial and complete dentures.
- ● The altered cast technique.

16

Overdentures

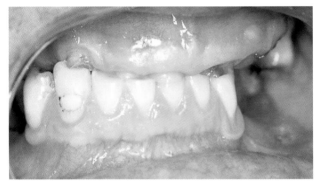

Fig. 16.1 The patient of Case 16 has worn his remaining upper anterior teeth to the gingival level.

Clinical details

This 65-year-old man requested replacement teeth as he was having increasing difficulty with chewing his food (Fig. 16.1). He noticed that his teeth had worn progressively over the last few years but now would like replacement. He complained that frequently after food and drink his stomach contents regurgitated into his mouth; this had been a problem for many years. He has managed to self-medicate for this by avoiding spicy and fatty foods and by taking over-the-counter anti-reflux drugs. What advice can you give and what is the cause of the tooth wear? What are the treatment options?

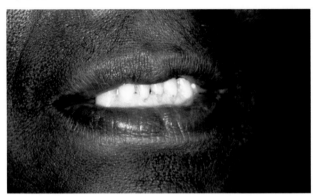

Fig. 16.2 The extra-oral appearance of the patient of Case 16. Despite the severe tooth wear, there has been little change in the vertical dimension.

Clinical observations

- The teeth are worn to the gingival margins with complete loss of the clinical crowns in the maxilla.
- There is no posterior support.
- As he closes into the intercuspal position his mandible slides forwards so that the upper and lower incisors are in contact.
- There is more tooth wear in the maxilla than in the mandible.
- There is little or no measurable loss of occlusal vertical dimension (Fig. 16.2).

Medical advice

The likely cause of the tooth wear is regurgitation of stomach juice due to an underlying reflux disease. It is not the responsibility or the duty of a dentist to give advice on how to control reflux. This patient should be directed towards the care of a gastroenterologist or his general medical practitioner for investigations or medication to control the regurgitation. A list of indications for which patients with reflux disease and dental erosion should be referred to a gastroenterologist is given in Box 16.1.

Box 16.1 Indications for which patients with significant dental erosion and symptoms of reflux should be referred to a gastroenterologist

Patients with palatal dental erosion whose symptoms of gastrointestinal reflux are interfering with their quality of life. Those who have been diagnosed with pathological reflux from 24-hour pH measurement would normally be offered medication. If patients are not prepared to consider medication at the outset of the investigations, perhaps the pH measurement is not indicated.

Patients who want to know the cause of their erosion, irrespective of the presence of symptoms and the potential for medication.

All other patients should be reviewed by their dentists; this review should include serial study casts, sometimes taken over a period of years. If erosion progresses despite restriction of dietary acids, the question of a 24-hour oesophageal pH test should be reconsidered.

Table 16.1 Options for managing tooth wear: advantages and disadvantages

Option	Advantages	Disadvantages
Monitoring study casts	Important when the patient is uncertain if restorations are needed If causes of the tooth wear have been eliminated there is no need for restorations This process can continue for many years	Balance needs to be achieved, if the tooth wear is slow, as to when restorations are needed; if the delay is too long there may be insufficient tooth tissue remaining for conventional restorations
Occlusal adjustment	Relatively simple in concept	Depends on the existing occlusal relationship; for some patients, extensive tooth preparation may be needed to create anterior space
Full mouth rehabilitation	Immediate result; no need for Dahl appliances and maintains vitality of teeth Composites are a conservative technique and cost-effective	Not conservative of tooth tissue with conventional crowns Costly if all teeth are crowned
Dahl appliance	Conserves vitality of tooth tissue Repositions gingival margins to original location May be considered to be reversible	Can have an unacceptable appearance if metal onlays are used Relatively long process, in the order of months Laboratory fees involved Contraindicated in partially dentate mouths
Surgical crown lengthening	Maintains existing vertical dimension Repositions gingival margin to a more apical location	Uncomfortable Surgically invasive May increase likelihood for root treatment May produce a poor interdental appearance The possibility of pulpal exposure after tooth preparation still exists
Elective devitalization	Particularly useful for extensively worn teeth with little crown height	Results in loss of vitality of teeth, decreasing their longevity Potential for root fractures increased; this is especially important for patients with attrition
Overdentures	Retains the teeth Preserves alveolar bone Relatively simple process	May need elective devitalization of teeth to prepare overdenture abutments The appearance can be compromised if prominent canine eminences are present

What is the cause of the tooth wear?

In the present case, there is probably a dual aetiology of erosion and attrition. The regurgitation of the stomach juice with its highly acidic contents has dissolved the enamel and dentine, but this has been exacerbated by a parafunctional habit. If attrition was the major cause, the tooth wear would be equal in both arches.

The slow wear has induced compensatory alveolar eruption which maintains the occlusal vertical dimension. The result is short clinical crowns without space for restorations.

What are the options for treatment?

Treatment of the worn dentition is not always indicated; Table 16.1 shows the range of treatment available.

● The upper jaw

If the tooth wear has progressed to an extent where little coronal tooth tissue remains, overdentures can be used to restore the appearance. The worn teeth can be electively devitalized and prepared level to the gingival margin. This is necessary where there is a limited amount of space between the arches for the denture bases. If the space is too narrow, the dentures are likely to fracture. Where a substantial space exists between the arches, it is possible to enhance the stability of the dentures either by leaving the worn teeth alone or by providing them with copings. Further retention can sometimes be gained by incorporating attachments.

Another possibility is elective root treatment of the remaining upper anterior teeth and restoration with post-retained crowns. The problems associated with post crowns in the presence of a parafunctional activity are that the posts may become loose, bend or fracture, or that the roots themselves may fracture longitudinally.

● The lower jaw

A conventional, tooth- and tissue-supported cobalt–chromium partial denture, or no prosthesis and maintain as a shortened dental arch.

What are the potential complications?

Canine eminence.
Parafunctional habit.
Tolerating the increased vertical dimension.
Fracture of the denture base.
Loss of vitality of the roots or teeth.
Caries.

● Canine eminence

If the patient's canine eminences are prominent, it may not be possible to extend the flange over these teeth because of undercut in relation to the path of insertion. A canine eminence is usually prominent in dentate patients. Any flange placed over this area may be difficult to make.

● Parafunctional habit

Patients with tooth wear caused by a parafunctional habit increases the risk of fracture of the base plate. A metal-backed base plate reduces this possibility but does not eliminate it.

● Tolerating the increased vertical dimension

Most patients with chronic tooth wear appear to tolerate increases in the vertical dimension without too much difficulty. It is suspected that the proprioceptors within the periodontal ligament provide a degree of feedback preventing overloading of the tissues. Edentulous patients have no such receptors, so reducing the feedback mechanism and tolerance to changes in the vertical dimension.

● Fracture of the denture base

If acrylic is finished close to the incisal edges of the teeth, fracture of the saddle area is possible. Metal backing increases the fracture resistance but additional clinical steps are needed when making the denture (Fig. 16.3).

● Loss of vitality of the roots or teeth

It is not always necessary to root-treat extensively worn teeth. The capacity of the pulp to adapt to change is often underestimated and therefore root treatments should only be carried out if the pulps lose their vitality. The vitality of the teeth should be assessed using conventional techniques.

● Caries

A common medium- to long-term complication of using teeth as overdenture abutments is dental caries. Combined with poor oral hygiene this can result in the eventual extraction of the tooth. Good oral hygiene supplemented with fluoride mouth washes may reduce the potential for caries to develop. There may also be complicating medical factors which tip the balance towards caries susceptibility. It is not uncommon for older patients to have multi-drug therapy which has the

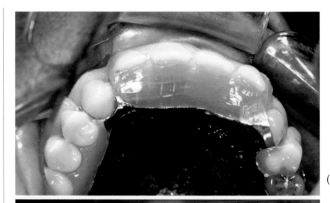

(a)

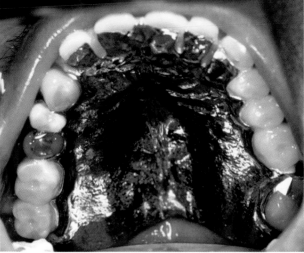

(b)

Fig. 16.3 (a) There is a risk of the saddle fracturing as the lower incisors contact the acrylic saddle area, even though a wire mesh has been used to strengthen this area. (b) The metal has been finished closer to the acrylic teeth, ensuring that the maximum stress from the opposing teeth is taken on the metal base.

side-effect of reducing salivary flow and thus removing its protective influence. Also it should not be forgotten that, as patients age, their ability to use a manual toothbrush may deteriorate and it would be sensible to advise them to start using an electric toothbrush.

Caries often develops around the access cavity margin. A glass ionomer can in theory provide protection against caries by the leaching of fluoride, but it will not overcome poor oral hygiene and a cariogenic diet. A traditional technique is to use gold post-retained copings to cover the access cavity and root surface of the abutment teeth. An advantage of this technique is that a precision attachment could be incorporated into the gold post to improve the retention of the denture.

What are the stages in making this partial denture?

Take primary impression and design the denture.
Take secondary impressions.
Record the occlusion.
Set up the anterior teeth in the right position.
Make and try the metal base.
Wax-up the denture.
Finish.

Primary impressions

Probably the most overlooked part of making partial or complete dentures is the primary impression. Often rushed and less than perfect impressions are accepted because the opportunity to improve the situation is left for the secondary stage. However, the problem with accepting an inadequate primary impression is that it is used to make the special tray and therefore errors made at this stage will be exaggerated in the secondary impression. The choice of material used in the primary impression varies between clinicians. If alginate is used, it is essential that the impression is cast within an hour, and preferably sooner, to reduce the potential for dimensional changes. If this is not possible, a silicone or polyether impression is more acceptable because these materials are more resistant to dimensional change. It is of great benefit to have a selection of stock trays and to use green stick compound to extend the periphery where required (not soft red wax, which distorts).

The interocclusal record

If a conformative approach is used to restore the partially dentate mouth, then the existing occlusal relationship must be accepted and the vertical dimension remains unchanged. Therefore, throughout the clinical stages, those teeth that had occlusal contacts with the opposing arch must have them at the fit of the denture. It is essential that rest seats, clasps and major or minor connectors should not interfere with the intercuspal position. Preparation of teeth for rest seats should provide sufficient interocclusal space for the rest and any minor connectors.

There are a variety of materials on the market for recording the interocclusal relationship of dentate patients and the choice will often be personal (Box 16.2). Generally, the material should be dimensionally stable, rigid, have a quick setting-time and be resistant to distortion. Wax combined with zinc oxide–eugenol or on its own can be useful, but the rigid silicone materials recently introduced can be particularly useful. Occlusal rims placed onto the edentulous ridge is the conventional method of recording the interocclusal relationship. The occlusal plane would normally be determined by the existing teeth and therefore be relatively straightforward. However, in some cases the occlusal plane needs to be changed prior to construction of the dentures. Crowning teeth, or on occasion extraction of teeth, will even out the occlusal plane, making it simpler to make the denture. When the occlusal plane is uneven and accepted without any adjustment, the denture can be difficult to make.

Provided that the interocclusal relationship is obvious, a technician may not need to be given a record, especially if there are few edentulous spaces, but it becomes essential when the casts cannot be located together easily. The clinician must also decide whether to use an articulator, and the indications used for fixed prosthodontics are equally relevant.

Anterior set-up

In most patients the set-up of the anterior teeth for cobalt–chromium partial dentures would be after the construction of the metal base. The anterior set-up should record the position of the incisal edge of the teeth, mid-line and the degree of support from the lips.

If the lower incisors contact the junction between the metal and acrylic on the saddle, there is a potential for this area to fracture. If the anterior set-up is recorded before the metal base is made, the position of the contact between the denture and the teeth can be more easily controlled to avoid this occurring.

Try-in of the metal base

One of the most important instructions to the technician should be to block out the undercuts on the model prior to making the metal base. Forgetting this can lead to prolonged chairside adjustment. Provided that the base is well made from an accurate impression, it should fit the patient with little adjustment. The base should be rigid, retentive and free of interferences. If the occlusion has not been recorded it should normally be done at this stage.

Try-in and fit of the denture

The final fit of the denture should be made so that both the patient and the dentist can insert and remove it easily.

What are the common eating disorders important in dentistry and their common medical complications?

Anorexia nervosa.
Bulimia nervosa.
Rumination.

Box 16.2 Taking interocclusal records

If it is possible to locate the intercuspal position (ICP) on hand-held study casts, an interocclusal record is unnecessary. In circumstances where the ICP is more difficult to identify on study casts, an interocclusal record of the teeth is necessary. One way is to draw the areas of contact between the upper and lower teeth on previously taken study casts. More commonly, a bite registration material is used to record the position of the prepared teeth in relation to the opposing jaw. Recently, silicone materials have been produced which set rapidly to produce a rigid material that can be carved with a sharp knife (e.g. Futar D; Kettenbach, Germany). Materials such as beauty wax or zinc oxide–eugenol pastes can be used, but these often prove to be too fragile and difficult to locate onto plaster or stone casts.

● Anorexia nervosa

This is a sociocultural disease affecting mainly white, upper middle-class women between the ages of 12 and 30 years. It is characterized by a disturbance of body image, presenting as an overwhelming desire to reduce weight to the detriment of health. This disease may begin abruptly as a single circumscribed episode or develop gradually over many months or even over a number of years. The prevalence of anorexia in men is not as well documented as in women and accurate figures are not known.

Anorexia is found in intelligent, highly motivated individuals, often with overprotective parents. A person with low self-esteem and compulsive behaviour who strives for perfection is more likely to develop the disease. It is a secretive disease which may pass through periods of exacerbations and quiescence. In some patients it is difficult to distinguish between anorexia and bulimia nervosa. Almost all anorexics deny the illness and refuse therapy and around 25% of the serious cases die from medical complications.

Medical aspects

Medical complications are induced by a combination of dietary restriction, reduced pleasure from food and self-induced vomiting. They include: amenorrhoea, caused by low levels of oestrogen in the blood, together with atrophic ovaries; and bradycardia, low pulse rates and arrhythmias, caused by a low metabolic rate. Treatment for the condition is generally unsatisfactory and most attempts are centred on group therapy. Efforts are directed at the person regaining physical health, reducing the symptoms and improving self-esteem, together with medication.

● Bulimia nervosa

Bulimia literally translated means 'ox hunger'. It affects a similar group of subjects as anorexia nervosa. Bulimics also have low self-esteem, but present as a slightly older age group than anorexics (20–30 years old); however, unlike anorexics, they are more out-going and amenable to therapy. Bulimics binge on vast amounts of food and then attempt to avoid weight gain by expelling it through self-induced vomiting. They tend to arrange schedules to allow sufficient time to binge and purge privately and food is often kept in secret places. Some may binge up to 20 times a day. These subjects may use laxatives and diuretics in an attempt to control weight fluctuations.

Medical aspects

The most significant medical problems are caused by changes in fluid and electrolyte balance resulting from persistent vomiting. These changes will affect the respiratory rate and cardiac output. Long-term sufferers will develop stomach dilation and gastro-oesophageal reflux disease.

● Rumination

Rumination can be defined as the deliberate regurgitation of food into the mouth from the stomach; some of the contents may be lost but the remainder is re-chewed and swallowed. It appears that ruminants are aware of the habit but may not necessarily be prepared to discuss the causes or seek advice.

Learning outcomes

- Risks of using overdentures.
- Interocclusal records for partial dentures.
- Common eating disorders related to dentistry.
- Indications for referral to a gastroenterologist for patients with dental erosion.
- Advantages and disadvantages of restoring worn teeth.
- Taking interocclusal records.

17

Edentulous maxilla

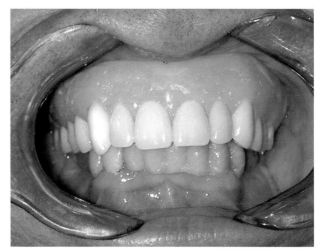

Fig. 17.1 Appearance of Case 17, edentulous maxilla.

Clinical details

This 60-year-old man had all his maxillary teeth extracted 8 years ago and has found the upper denture increasingly unstable (Fig. 17.1). A denture was provided immediately after the last teeth were extracted and was replaced 6 months later. The existing denture has been replaced twice. The lower anterior teeth are provisionally restored with a bridge, but are clinically sound, caries-free and not periodontally involved. The medical history is clear.

Clinical observations

■ A fibrous (flabby) edentulous ridge opposes the lower anterior teeth.

■ The lower edentulous ridge extends distal to the canines and is extensively resorbed.

What additional information do you require?

The peripheral extensions of the existing denture.
The degree of mobility of the fibrous ridge.

● The peripheral extensions of the existing denture

The extensions of the existing denture need to be assessed. If the denture does not have full extensions into the buccal sulcus or around the maxillary tuberosity, its retention will be compromised. The other area to investigate is the post dam to see if it extends up to the vibrating line (junction of hard and soft palate).

● The degree of mobility of the fibrous ridge

It will be difficult to overcome the mobility of the fibrous ridge. However, the denture base overlying the fibrous ridge needs to be well supported and the buccal flange should be made to the full depth of the sulcus. This concept is difficult to achieve practically.

What impression technique could you use to record the fibrous (flabby) ridge?

The clinical relevance of either a mucostatic or a mucocompressive impression technique for recording a fibrous (flabby) ridge is probably minor. The difficulty lies with the mobility of the fibrous ridge and the impact it has on the support for the denture. A well-extended two-part special tray can be used with zinc oxide–eugenol or a silicone impression material. The peripheral extensions are recorded by the main part of the special tray but a window is left open overlying the fibrous ridge. At the same time as the zinc oxide–eugenol (or silicone) is setting, the window overlying the fibrous ridge is coated with the impression material and a sectional part of the tray attached to support the flowing zinc oxide–eugenol. A flabby ridge can also be surgically removed.

What are the options for treatment?

Well-fitting replacement conventional denture.
Implant-supported prosthesis, either with an:
    Overdenture with two fixtures placed in the canine region or a
    Fixed bridge with 4–6 fixtures.

A well-fitting conventional denture may overcome the difficulties presented by the unstable complete denture. However, some patients continue to find these dentures difficult to tolerate and an implant-supported solution may need considering. The most important requirement for implants is sufficient height and width of bone. Without this, bone augmentation may be necessary, which will substantially increase the cost. A cost-effective solution is an implant-supported complete overdenture using two fixtures in the canine region and precision attachments in the fit surface of the denture.

Learning outcomes

● Complications of upper complete dentures opposed by teeth.

● Recognition and the management of a flabby ridge.

18

Complete dentures

Clinical details

A patient, 70 years of age, presents himself at your surgery seeking the construction of a new set of dentures (Fig. 18.1). He reports that his current dentures were fitted 6 months previously at the same time that his last few remaining upper and lower teeth were extracted. Previously he had, for many years, successfully worn upper and lower acrylic resin partial dentures. Progressive tooth loss had resulted from chronic periodontitis and root caries. He has many problems with his new dentures, not least of which is his inability to wear them for more than a few minutes at a time. He finds both the upper and lower dentures have become progressively loose and he suffers soreness under the lower denture base. What are the likely causes of your patient's complaints and what steps would you take to prevent their repetition?

Clinical observations

- Substantial resorption of the alveolar ridges; the pattern of resorption is irregular, resulting in uneven ridges.
- Fibrous changes have taken place in the anterior maxilla; in the posterior mandible the ridge form is sharp.
- The dentures lack retention and stability.
- The base extension is inadequate and there are gaps between areas of the mucosa and the denture base.
- A small gap is visible between the left premolar and molar teeth when the right side teeth are in contact.
- Excursive movements of the jaw readily displace the dentures.

What are the potential complicating factors?

Achieving a satisfactory transition from partial dentures, retained by a few teeth, to complete dentures is, for a number of reasons, often unsatisfactory (see below).

Making an accurate and correctly extended impression of the denture-bearing areas is complicated by the very presence of the teeth that are to be replaced. This is particularly so if these teeth have been affected by periodontal disease, which often results in long clinical crowns, drifting and tilting.

With a few exceptions, stock impression trays are not designed to cater for the transition between the natural and complete dentures.

What are the stages in constructing complete immediate-replacement dentures?

The impression.
Special trays.
Jaw relation record.
The try-in stage.

● The impression

Stock trays need to be modified by adding a malleable material, such as impression compound or impression putty, to those parts of the tray that are to record the edentulous areas (Fig. 18.2). These additions give support to the wash material, usually alginate, particularly in the border areas of the impression. Despite careful modification of stock trays, it is rarely possible to achieve an impression of sufficient accuracy and correct extension.

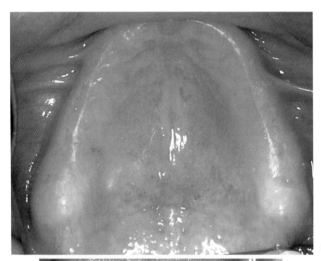

(a)

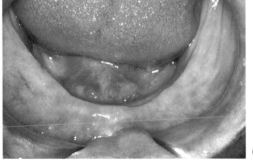

(b)

Fig. 18.1 Edentulous ridges of Case 18.

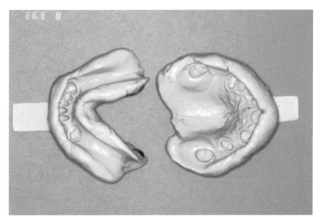

Fig. 18.2 Well-extended primary impressions showing all the major anatomical features.

For this reason, the model that is made from this 'primary' impression is best used to construct a special (or custom-made) tray.

● Special trays

The main advantages of special trays over stock trays is that the former can be extended correctly into the sulci and made with a uniform space between the inner tray surface and the oral tissues. This reduces distortion when alginate is used as the impression material.

The clinical handling of special trays is not without its difficulties. Trays can be quite large and awkward to manoeuvre into the mouth. Loaded with alginate, they can be difficult to position and align correctly. This failure often results in distorted impressions of the buccal sulci and teeth or soft tissue touching the tray. Once taken, a decision has to be made as to whether or not the impression is acceptable. Unless more than one tray has been made, it cannot be put aside while a second impression is taken to see if it can be improved upon.

● Jaw relation record

Ideally, the jaw relation should be recorded at the correct vertical dimension and with the temporomandibular joints in the retruded position. Recording the jaw relation is often complicated by the presence of teeth. A few teeth remaining in each arch often serve to guide the mandible during its final path of closure into a protrusive or lateral position. This may be accompanied by a powerful postural habit that makes manipulating the mandible around the terminal hinge axis particularly challenging.

● The try-in stage

As the try-in stage has to be done prior to the extractions, clearly only the existing edentulous areas can be restored with denture teeth set in wax. Although this does have limitations, it does serve to verify that the correct shade and mould of prosthetic tooth has been chosen.

Verification of tooth position can be more difficult or sometimes quite impossible. Drifting of the remaining teeth may prevent the correct positioning of the prosthetic teeth until the natural teeth are sectioned from the working model prior to final wax-up and flasking. As a result it may not, for example, be possible to arrange the teeth for try-in with the correct centre line. In such a case, it would be necessary to accurately mark on the wax flange the correct position of the centre lines so that the teeth can be re-set before the dentures are completed.

The try-in is also the stage at which the jaw relation record is checked for accuracy, in both its vertical and horizontal dimensions. As with the jaw relation record stage, however, the presence of teeth can make this procedure difficult.

The removal of the remaining teeth and the consequent effect upon proprioception has been shown to be accompanied by a reduction of the rest vertical dimension. For this reason, it has been advocated that an arbitrary reduction of 1–2 mm in the occlusal vertical dimension be made when all the teeth are set-up in wax prior to flasking.

Delivery of the new complete dentures at the time of the extraction of the remaining teeth will only be successful if great care and attention is taken at all the clinical and construction stages. The patient must understand that the dentures may require adjustment in the early stages to relieve any sore spots and that, as healing and tissue re-modelling proceed, temporary re-lining will be necessary. After a few weeks, a self-curing acrylic resin relining material may have to be applied and it should be expected that the dentures will need to be re-made or re-lined after 6–9 months.

What is meant by balanced occlusion and articulation for complete dentures?

The Glossary of Prosthodontic Terms defines balanced occlusion as 'simultaneous contacts of the occluding surfaces on both sides of the mouth, in various jaw positions'. This is not a particularly helpful definition. For the complete denture case, it is more useful to understand the difference between a 'balanced occlusion' and a 'balanced articulation'. It is also essential to understand that the presence of a bolus of food between the teeth completely negates the concept of 'balanced occlusion'. It is understood, however, that there are numerous 'empty mouth' tooth contacts taking place every hour. It is when these occur that the concept of 'balance' becomes relevant.

Balanced occlusion Bilateral even contact between the upper and lower denture teeth at the selected intercuspal position. This is a static position.

Balanced articulation Bilateral even contact between the upper and lower denture teeth in lateral and protrusive positions of the mandible.

Constructing dentures with a balanced occlusion and articulation is highly desirable because:

Occlusal forces are transmitted evenly to the alveolar ridges, thereby reducing the risk of soreness of the alveolar mucosa.

Empty mouth tooth contact reinforces retention rather than acting to destabilize the dentures.

The difference between a balanced occlusion and a balanced articulation is that, with the latter, the upper and lower denture teeth should be in even contact when the jaws occlude in protrusive and lateral positions. This imparts greater stability to the dentures when they come into contact with each other.

To achieve a balanced occlusion requires that an accurate record of the jaw relationship be taken at a chosen vertical dimension of occlusion with the mandible at the retruded contact position (RCP). This record can then be transferred to a plane-line articulator for the trial set-up of the denture teeth.

To achieve a balanced articulation requires the use of an adjustable articulator set to mimic, as closely as possible, the movements of the jaw. A face-bow record is required to make records of the mandible in RCP and lateral excursions. With these records, movements of the articulator will replicate the movements of the jaw. Denture teeth set up in balance on the articulated casts should remain in balance when transferred to the mouth.

Learning outcomes

- Stability and support for complete dentures.
- Construction of immediate complete dentures.
- Differences between balanced occlusion and articulation for complete dentures.

19

Failed crown and bridge

Clinical details

A 19-year-old man presents to your surgery requesting dental treatment (Fig. 19.1). He appears well motivated and a series of appointments are made for his routine treatment. The patient is otherwise fit and well. He is about to leave home for a university degree course lasting 3 years. How would you manage this case?

Clinical observations

- There are a number of carious teeth.
- The patient lost LL5 and LL6 3 years ago due to caries.
- Another dentist started the root treatment on the lower right first molar.
- The patient's diet was highly cariogenic. He was drinking tea with sugar every few hours and snacking with biscuits throughout the day. This had been a habit for a number of years. Despite being aware that this could be damaging his teeth, he was at that time unwilling to change his lifestyle.
- Bite-wings were taken to diagnose the caries accurately. The vitality of the lower left second molar was tested with an electric pulp tester and found to give a vital response.

- There is no evidence of periodontal disease and the probing depths are all within normal limits. There was plaque present interproximally between a number of teeth.

Complicating factors

There are no obvious complicating factors.

What are the options for treatment?

The first aim of treatment is to stabilize the caries and complete the endodontics on the lower right first molar. Prevention with dietary advice and oral hygiene instruction should be started immediately and reinforced at regular intervals. Patients remember only part of the information given to them at each visit and therefore reinforcement has been shown to be particularly helpful in assisting them to become dentally aware. The patient should be shown how to use floss and advised how to use disclosing tablets to show the areas where cleaning has not been efficient.

The bite-wing radiographs showed caries on the occlusal and mesial surfaces of the LR6, recurrent caries on the LL7 and extensive caries on the UL5. Elsewhere, there was evidence of early caries, just into the enamel, on a number of teeth.

The endodontics on the LR6 needs to be replaced and completed and a coronal seal placed either with amalgam or composite.

If the caries was stabilized, the missing lower left teeth could be replaced with either a bridge or an implant. The design might be a conventional bridge retainer on the LL7 and possibly the same on the LL4 using a fixed-movable design. Alternatively, a hybrid bridge using a conventional retainer on the molar and a minimal preparation bridge retainer on the premolar is possible, again using a fixed-movable design. The movable joint should be placed distal to the premolar. Alternatively, two fixtures could be used to replace the missing teeth without the need to use either teeth as abutments.

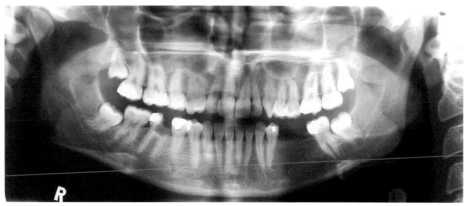

Fig. 19.1 A panoral view of Case 19 at the time of first presentation.

FIVE YEARS LATER

Clinical details

The patient presents to you again some 5 years later, after having left your practice before you could start the treatment (Fig. 19.2). He has just returned to your area after completing his degree course at university. How would you manage the problem?

Clinical observations

- There is now widespread caries; the UL8 is unrestorable.
- A number of teeth have periapical lesions. The root treatments on the UL7 and LR7 are inadequate.
- There is a periapical radiolucency associated with both roots on the LR7, which is inadequately obturated; the tooth has a poor prognosis.
- There is no root treatment associated with the post crown on the UL3. Similarly, there is no root treatment present on the UR5, which is further compromised by an ill-fitting crown and a deficiency beneath the crown which is filled with cement. The tooth has a poor prognosis.
- A periapical radiograph indicates that the UL3 has recurrent caries under the post crown and has a very poor prognosis. There are also periapical lesions on the UL4 and UL5.
- The root canal on the UL4 appears to be sclerosed. There are at least two roots that have disto-apical curves. This tooth will be difficult to root-treat. The

UL5 has a post crown without an adequate root treatment.
- At some time over the past 3 years the LR6 has been extracted.

What might be your provisional treatment?

The most important factor is to determine why the patient is not returning to the dentist who provided the original treatment. With any potential litigation, the more information from the patient and original dentist is needed before treatment is started. In this case it would be beneficial to seek medicolegal advice from your professional association before starting treatment. You must also attempt to discover if there were any accentuating circumstances that might have affected treatment. Finally, it is imperative that you establish that the patient is willing to complete treatment under your care considering his recent history.

The next phase is to again attempt to stabilize the disease. Dietary advice is needed, together with an improvement of oral hygiene. The poor dentition may be compounded by the patient's lack of cooperation.

The UL3 and UR4 need investigating to establish if they are restorable. The crowns need removing and the extent of the caries established in the root before further treatment. A provisional replacement should be available if the crowns cannot be re-cemented. Therefore, in the early phase of treatment, a removable acrylic denture should be made with replacements for the UL3 and UR4. This would allow sufficient time for initial resorption of the ridge to occur prior to a more long-term replacement.

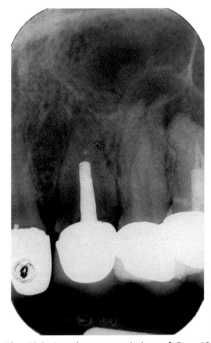
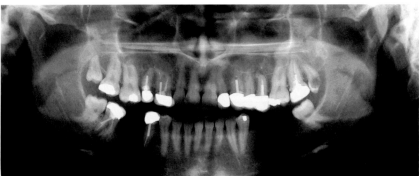

Fig. 19.2 Another panoral view of Case 19, taken 5 years later after the patient had been to university, together with a periapical radiograph of the canine.

Both teeth have a very poor prognosis and are likely to be extracted.

The status of the UL4 needs a similar evaluation. Is it within your capability to root treat? If not, is there a specialist available to carry out the treatment and is the patient able to afford the cost? Also, what is the prognosis of the tooth after the root treatment, considering the extent of the sclerosis?

The post-retained crown in the UL5 needs removing. This can be achieved with a combination of ultrasonics, with copious irrigation, to break the cement lute and leverage from a dental instrument or a post remover. However, care should be taken and the patient warned of the risk of root fracture when posts are removed. If the cement was an adhesive one it is likely that the post would be difficult to remove; more importantly, if the post de-cemented, the adhesive lute would be very difficult to remove from the walls of the root canal.

The UL7 also needs investigating to establish if it can be saved. The root treatments are inadequate, they are poorly obturated and do not reach the apical 1–2 mm. You must decide if you are capable of re-root-treating this tooth.

Potentially, the UL3, UL4, UL5, UR5 LR7, UL8 and possibly the UL7 may need extracting.

During this initial phase of treatment it will be possible for you to assess the motivation of the patient and you should then be able to assess what definitive treatment may be possible.

What are the options for definitive treatment?

Implants.
Fixed or removable prostheses.
A combination of all three.

The assessment made earlier about the UL3, UL4 and UL5 is important. If the patient is willing to fund implants, the loss of these teeth is probably prudent in that the cost of specialist endodontics combined with crowns and the difficulty of the treatment might mean that implants would be a better long-term prospect. Two fixtures placed in the canine and second premolar region could retain a fixed bridge replacing all three teeth. If the LR7 was also extracted, two or three fixtures, depending on the available space, could replace the missing teeth on both sides of the

mandible. However, the position of the inferior dental bundle needs to be assessed prior to their placement.

The missing UR5 could be replaced with a bridge. The relatively poor prognosis of the UR4 might suggest that this tooth is not used in the restoration. Either a conventional or minimal preparation bridge using the UR6 abutment as a simple cantilever is therefore a possibility.

If the patient chooses not to have implants, removable dentures would be a safer option than conventional bridges in the mandible. If the LR7 proved to be asymptomatic, it would still have a poor prognosis and not be suitable as a bridge abutment. Therefore, a denture on the right side and effectively on the left side would be the only option. If this tooth were lost, a conventional bridge from the last standing tooth to the premolars would, in theory, be a possibility, but the prognosis in a patient of this age would be poor. To complicate matters, the LR5 has a post-retained crown which would compromise a bridge, and its prognosis would not be improved by double-abutting with the LR4.

In the maxilla, it is crucial to determine the restorability of the UL3, UL4 and UL5. If they are unrestorable, the only feasible option would be a partial denture incorporating the UR5. If the UL3 were extracted and either the UL4 or UL5 or both were restored, a conventional bridge replacing one or two teeth could replace the missing ones. However, the cost of specialist treatment might exceed the cost of implants and make them a more feasible option.

In failing dentitions with multiple crowns and bridges it is often sensible to take a pragmatic or cautious approach. If implants are not possible for funding reasons, a conservative approach to the mouth is imperative. It may be prudent to accept less than perfect restorations or endodontics for the short to medium term, provided the teeth are asymptomatic and caries-free and those with active lesions are either extracted or the restorations replaced. It is relatively common after life-style changes to alter dietary habits and increase the risk of caries.

Learning outcomes

● The importance of maintaining oral hygiene and dietary advice after life-style changes.

20

Planning treatment around failed crowns

Clinical details

This 40-year-old man presents requesting replacement anterior teeth and routine treatment (Fig. 20.1). He is medically fit and well and has recently moved to your area. The post retained crowns support an anterior bridge which was 8 years old. The bridge initially became loose and only recently came out. He had not been to see a dentist for 3 years. How would you assess this patient and what are your options?

Clinical observations

- There are fractured posts in the UR3 and UR1.
- The UR2, UL1 and UL2 are missing in the upper anterior region. In addition, the LR6 is missing, the LL5 is missing and LL6 has drifted mesially and is the last standing tooth on that side.
- The LR4 and LR5 are both root-treated but do not have coronal seals. There is a large mesial periapical radiolucency surrounding the distal aspect of the LR4 root, which is poorly obturated. There is no draining periodontal pocket communicating with the oral cavity.

- Elsewhere, caries was not detected clinically or on bite-wing radiographs.
- The periodontal condition is good.

What are the options for provisional treatment?

The first phase of treatment is to establish if the fractured posts in the UR3 and UR1 can be removed. The most successful method is to use ultrasonic vibration to loosen or weaken the cement lute and then use a post remover to extract the post. However, both posts have fractured below the gingival margin and it might be difficult to use a post remover. The other option is to use the Masseran trephine kit in conjunction with ultrasonic vibration. Once the cement has been disrupted the Masseran drills can be threaded around the post and extracted. If the post cannot be removed the teeth will be unrestorable and need extracting.

For the interim period, a removable partial denture would replace the missing teeth while allowing continuation of treatment to the teeth.

The LR5 needs an adequate coronal seal. This tooth could be used as a retainer for a bridge replacing the LR6. Therefore, the prognosis of this tooth needs to be established prior to this being started.

The LR4 has a large periapical lesion on the distal surface of the root which remains asymptomatic. The root treatment will need replacing and then reviewing to ensure the radiolucency resolves.

What are the options for definitive treatment?

If the posts were successfully removed and the endodontics repeated on both teeth, a conventional bridge could replace the missing teeth. The possibilities are:

- A fixed-fixed bridge using a conventional crown on the UL3 and a post-retained crown on the UR1. A

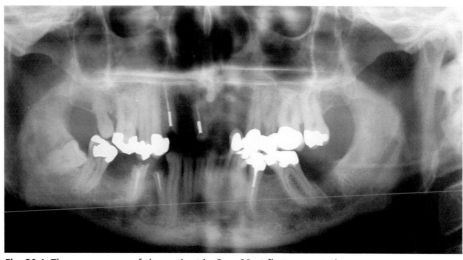

Fig. 20.1 The appearance of the patient in Case 20 at first presentation.

post-retained crown on the UR3 could support a cantilever pontic replacing the UR2. This design, however, does have the potential to place high torsional forces on the abutment tooth and should only be contemplated in selected cases.

- A fixed-fixed bridge from canine to canine incorporating the UR1. However, if it failed around the UR1, this would mean the total loss of the bridge, unlike the option above, which has a degree of retrievability.
- If the post could not be removed from the UR3 and UR1, a bridge would no longer be a feasible option and either implants or dentures would have to be used to replace the teeth once they were extracted.

Perhaps three fixtures would be needed to replace the missing teeth: one each in the UR3 and UR2 region and another in UL2 region.

- A conventional fixed-movable bridge in the lower right quadrant from the LR7 to the LR5. Alternatively, a single tooth implant could replace the missing tooth. On the left side, the missing LL7 and LL8 could be left unrestored.

Learning outcomes

● Planning crowns and bridges around failing restorations.

21

Bone augmentation

Clinical details

One month ago this patient had augmentation of the maxilla with bone taken from the iliac crest for implants (Fig. 21.1). He is medically fit and well, but smokes fewer than five cigarettes a day. He is expecting implants in the maxilla and in the mandible to replace his missing teeth. When will you arrange for the implants and how will you assess which type of fixture is needed? What will be your choice of abutment?

Clinical observations

- The patient has a mild class II division 1 incisal relationship with an overjet of 5 mm with his existing dentures.
- He has had dentures for 5 years but they have become increasingly unstable and he has gradually developed a debilitating gag reflex.
- There was sufficient bone in the mandible, but earlier investigations indicated that this was not the case in the maxilla and he needed bone augmentation. This was achieved by taking bone from the iliac crest, securing it with mini-plates and screws some 4 weeks prior to the radiograph.

- Immediately after the surgery he had a pronounced limp, but this has improved over the past couple of weeks.

What are the potential complicating factors?

Resorption.

Incisal relationship.

Ideally, loading should not occur within 3 months, but some surgeons recommend much shorter periods because of the likelihood of bone resorption. The eventual decision to start the placement of the implants will depend on the presence of any postoperative complications, the amount of bone replaced and the radiographic evidence.

● Resorption

Bone augmentation can be resorbed soon after surgery. Smoking may influence the success of the augmentation and also of the implants. Ideally, patients should stop smoking prior to any implant surgery, but are often reluctant to do so. About 95% of implants placed in the lower anterior region succeed, whilst the figure is a little lower in the maxilla at 85–90% over 5 years. Like teeth, a process called peri-implantitis, which is not unlike periodontitis, can resorb the bone surrounding the implant. Normally, this occurs evenly around the circumference of the fixture as the bone recedes apically, unlike periodontitis where the bone loss is more irregular. A convenient measure of the activity is the number of threads exposed by the disease. The immediate postoperative radiograph is a good reference point with which to compare the progression of disease. Commonly, in the first few years, bone is lost around the first thread of the implant, but, if it continues, the implant may be compromised. If the disease progresses, the implant is supported by less and less bone, allowing damaging lateral forces to increase the potential for fracture of the metal implant or increase the mobility to such an extent that failure is inevitable.

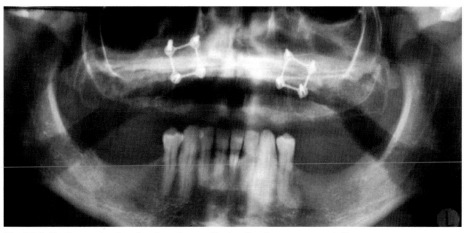

Fig. 21.1 Radiograph of patient postoperatively after bone augmentation.

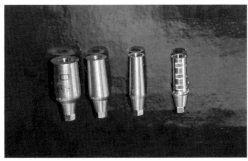

Fig. 21.2 Single-tooth metal prepable abutments at (from the left) 7.0 mm, 5.5 mm and 4.5 mm (Astra Tech, Molndal, Sweden). The abutment on the far right is an example of the Cast-To system (see Fig. 21.3).

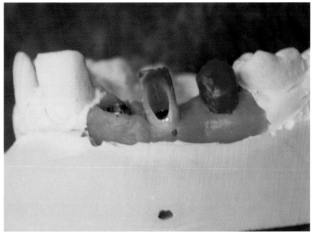

Fig. 21.3 The Astra Cast-To implant system. This involves placing a plastic burn-out sleeve over the abutment, which is subsequently waxed-up to form the crown and then cast in gold for a cemented bridge abutment. (Courtesy of Mr Safiullah and Suzanne Street.)

Peri-implantitis, like periodontal disease, is prevented with good oral hygiene. Probing depths should not exceed 4 mm without bleeding and there should be an absence of pus or swelling around the abutment. There should also be no other symptoms, such as tenderness around the implant site, mobility or swelling. Provided the patient's oral hygiene is good, there is no reason to suppose that the implant will not survive many years of use.

● **Incisal relationship**

A decision must be reached whether to conform to the patient's existing incisal relationship or place the implants further palatally to achieve a class I relationship. To do this, the existing dentures should be evaluated by both dentist and patient. If the patient is satisfied with the existing incisal relationship, the easiest management would be to place the abutments in the same position as the teeth and use the denture to make a template for the surgery. However, if the orientation is changed to produce a class I incisal relationship, a change in the angulation of the fixtures might mean that there is insufficient height and width of bone in which to place the implants. When the orientation of the fixture is not ideal, some flexibility can be accommodated by prepable abutments. These can be prepared by either the dentist or technician to create an ideal emergence angle for the crown (Figs 21.2 and 21.3).

If the original tooth position is chosen, the existing denture can also be used during the diagnostic evaluation of the quantity of bone. Metal tags can be attached to the denture in the potential fixture sites and the amount of bone assessed with radiographs. The radio-opaque tags or balls are superimposed over the bone to allow the clinician to visualize the intended position of the fixture and the restoration. If the tooth position is changed, then a new diagnostic set-up needs to be made. Once the position of the implants has been decided, a stent can be made to guide the surgeon during placing of the implants.

FOLLOWING IMPLANT PLACEMENT

The implants were placed 6 months after the sinus graft and equally spaced along the maxilla (Fig. 21.4).

How do you assess the optimum number of implants and how do you choose their position?

Orientation of implants.
Number of implants.
Choice of abutment.
Choice of impression and impression technique.
Securing the abutment.

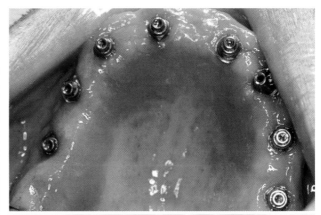

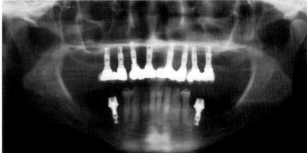

Fig. 21.4 The implants were placed in the approximate tooth position. Note the rather central position of the mid-line abutment. This will make the construction of the restoration difficult. Ideally, the fixtures should have been placed to one side of the mid-line to give the technician space for a symmetrical appearance.

Box 21.1 Typical characteristics of fixtures

Implant length This varies between manufacturers, but the most commonly used is 8–15 mm long with a range of 6–20 mm.

Implant diameter Most are 4 mm in diameter with a thread pitch of about 0.6 mm and a range of 3.25–6.5 mm. Those with diameters of less than 3.25 mm are generally too narrow and may have insufficient strength.

Implant shape Most current fixtures are solid rather than hollow, as the latter design has an increased susceptibility to fracture. The Frialit has a tooth-like shape, being narrower at the apical end; others, such as the Branemark, are parallel-sided (Fig. 21.8a). The Astra Tech has a widened collar but a parallel-sided trunk (Fig. 21.8b).

● Orientation of implants

The orientation of the implant should be determined pre-operatively so that the best position is chosen for the restorations. Sometimes this is not possible as the site has less bone than was predicted from the pre-operative diagnostic tests, so the fixture is placed in an area surrounded by the greatest amount of bone. Angled abutments can overcome slight modifications in position of the fixture but they have limitations. More recently, prepable abutments have been introduced which give the same degree of flexibility as angled abutments (Figs 21.2 and 21.3); they are more adaptable but can only have cemented restorations. Implants should not be placed in positions that might compromise vital structures, such as the inferior dental bundle, nasal or sinus cavities and adjacent teeth, but in the ideal position for the teeth.

● Number of implants

There is little guidance to indicate the most appropriate number of implants. Generally, for one or two missing teeth, a single implant is needed, whereas for a greater number of missing teeth the selection will depend on the size of the natural teeth and the length of the edentulous span (see Boxes 21.1 and 21.2). For an edentulous maxilla at least five should be placed, but in this case eight were used (Fig. 21.4). Too many implants will crowd the site and may compromise the appearance of the restoration; but, more importantly, at least 1–2 mm of bone should be left between fixtures to allow sufficient space to attach the abutments and for access during cleaning. Most operators would prefer to avoid linking teeth to implants because natural teeth move slightly within bone and implants do not, although some studies have shown favourable results.

● Choice of abutment

After stage 2 surgery, the implant-healing caps are removed and the amount of soft tissue above the implant is measured. At this stage, either the abutment is selected or a head of fixture impression taken so that an abutment can be selected in the laboratory. There is considerable choice of design and type of material from the manufacturers of the abutments. The choice will to a large extent depend upon the clinician's own experience and whether the restoration is to be cemented or screw-retained.

● Choice of impression and impression technique

Either the abutment can be attached to the fixture and an impression taken of its location, or the healing cap is removed and an impression taken of the head of the fixture. The first method involves choosing the type of abutment at the chairside before taking the impression; thus the dentist is committed to a particular abutment early in the decision-making process. The latter method allows both the set-up to be assessed and the best abutment to be chosen in the laboratory (Figs 21.5 and 21.6).

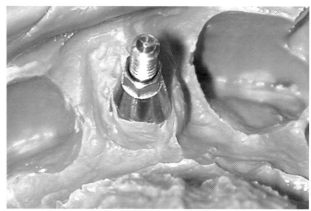

Fig. 21.5 Impressions for implants are usually taken using the head of fixture technique. The clinician records the position of the fixture with an impression replica screwed into the head of the fixture with a guide pin. The impression is cast using a laboratory replica of the fixture. The chosen abutment is screwed onto this and the crown made using a suitable gold or ceramic cap. The example shown is an Astra single-tooth implant. (Courtesy of Mr Safiullah and Suzanne Street.)

Box 21.2 Some common implant manufacturers

Branemark (Nobel Biocare, Sweden)

Astra Tech (Sweden)

Straumann (Switzerland)

Frialit (Friadent, Germany)

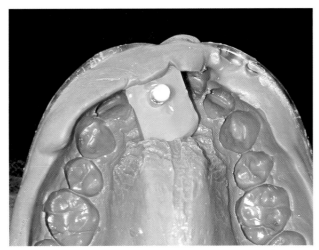

Fig. 21.6 The laboratory replica is attached to the abutment and a pink-coloured silicone poured around them to mimic the gingival tissues. The gingival mask is used to assist the technician when making the crown to record the depth of the sulcus and help construct the emergence profile. (Courtesy of Mr Safiullah and Suzanne Street.)

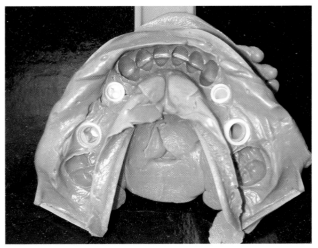

Fig. 21.7 An alternative technique to that shown in Fig. 21.6 is to use impression copings to record the position of the abutment. This relies upon the coping being fully seated within the impression material rather than being screwed down; otherwise, inaccuracies will develop during the making of the crown. This is an example of the Straumann solid abutment system (Straumann/ITI, Switzerland), where the bridge will be cemented over the abutments. (Courtesy of Mr Safiullah and Suzanne Street.)

Both impression techniques usually involve metal copings (Fig. 21.7). The area overlying the fixtures is cut away on the impression tray so that after the impression the transfer copings perforate through the top of the tray, providing sufficient access to loosen the screws attaching it to the fixture. The pins are removed, leaving the copings to record the position of the head of the fixture. The laboratory technician and the clinician can then assess, in the comfort of the laboratory, the most appropriate type, material and angulation of the abutment. The impression material needs to be sufficiently rigid to record the position of the implant but also resilient enough to be removed over undercuts.

● Securing the abutment

Once the abutment has been chosen it needs to be secured to the fixture by a screw. Care must be taken to ensure that the abutment is fully down and contacting the fixture; to check this, a radiograph is normally taken immediately after location and prior to the final tightening of the abutment (Fig. 21.8).

Treatment of Case 21

The full arch bridge was split into three parts to simplify the bridge construction (Fig. 21.9a). Two posterior bridges and one anterior bridge were supported by eight fixtures; a further two single-tooth implants were used in the mandibular (Fig. 21.9b). Their distal inclination made the seating and positioning of the abutments difficult (Fig. 21.9c).

What types of bone grafting are possible?

Autologous: minor, moderate, major.
Alloplastic.

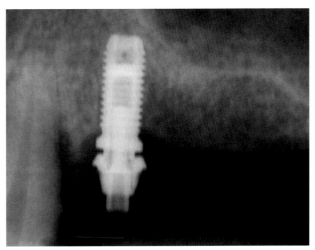

(a)

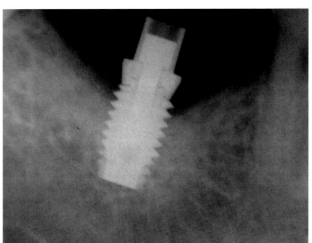

(b)

Fig. 21.8 Radiographs showing an abutment that is incorrectly seated onto the fixture (a) and one that is properly seated (b).

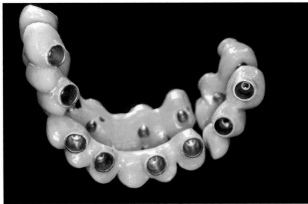

(a)

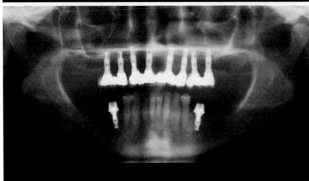

(b)

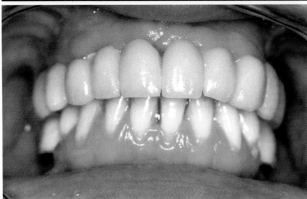

(c)

Fig. 21.9 The definitive treatment for Case 21. (a) The three-part bridge. (b) Radiograph showing the positioning of the implants. (c) The finished result, with the implant-retained bridge screwed into position; the less than ideal appearance reflects the difficulty of the case and the original compromised amount of bone.

● Autologous grafts

Minor bone loss

Often after extractions, and especially after minor oral surgery, bone may be lost from the buccal plate, resulting in small defects. If a fixture is placed in the same area it may not be totally surrounded or embedded in bone. Provided the amount of bone loss is minor, this may not be a problem. The excess from the surgical site created during the fixture placement can fill minor bone defects. Additional bone can be harvested from the central core of the drill that was used during the implant surgery. This could be supplemented with guided-tissue regeneration.

Moderate bone loss

For more advanced cases of alveolar bone loss, the relatively small amount of bone gained from the surgical site

is insufficient and thus more bone is needed. Typically, this can be harvested from the chin or retromolar region and can be secured to the new site with mini-screws and plates. Another way to gain additional bone is to split and expand the buccolingual alveolar bone with osteotomes and, provided the bone is not brittle and the blood supply is adequate, the infill should provide more bone around the fixture.

Advanced bone loss

The most common area needing additional bone is the posterior maxilla distal to the canines. Pre-operatively, the maxillary sinus can be closely approximated to the alveolar ridge, leaving insufficient bone for implants. Bone can be added and secured with mini-plates and screws into the maxillary sinus through a Caldwell-Luc procedure. For more advanced cases, a Le Fort I type osteotomy will create more bone, but increases the surgical risks. The most common harvesting site is the iliac crest. Increasing the complexity of implant surgery not only increases the risk of failure but also the cost.

● Alloplastic grafts

These materials are usually composed of hydroxyapatite, tricalcium phosphate or active bioglass. They provide a framework for autogenous bone to infiltrate and eventually strengthen. The hydroxyapatite can be dispensed in porous or dense blocks from human (allografts) or bovine (xenografts) sources, both of which may have potential infective risks.

What types of abutment are possible?

Single-tooth abutments.
Bridge abutments.
Overdenture abutments.

● Single-tooth abutments

The most important criterion for single teeth is an anti-rotational device incorporated into the fixture head (Fig. 21.10). Many manufacturers use hexagonal shapes within the abutment head and the fixture. The hexagonal shape prevents rotation of the abutment relative to the fixture, preventing loosening of the implant. The abutment margin should be placed 2 mm subgingivally to produce optimum aesthetics. The crown may be made from metal fused to porcelain or an all-porcelain crown such as Procera (Nobel Biocare, Sweden) can be used. Some manufacturers have introduced ceramic abutments in an effort to improve the translucency of the restoration. In theory, these abutments have very high tensile strengths, but their long-term success has yet to be fully appraised.

A fixture should be placed in the ideal location for the crown. Sometimes the ideal position and the area of most bone are not the same, in which case the position is more important than the bone which can be grafted.

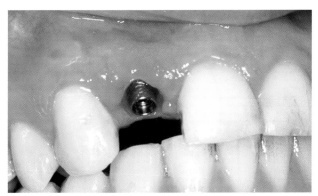

Fig. 21.10 Single-tooth implant (Astra) with an anti-rotational design to prevent rotation. The hexagonal shape is just visible.

A diagnostic wax-up of the proposed location of the restoration will show where the abutments should be placed. If the position is beyond the scope of the standard abutment, another type will need selecting. Angled abutments (either 15° or 30°) or, more commonly, prepable abutments, can provide a limited degree of flexibility, but they have limitations. Either the laboratory can prepare the abutment or the clinician can do it in the mouth. The eventual shape and position should give the restoration the best appearance. Each manufacturer provides implants with individual qualities, which make their product unique, and the choice usually depends on the experience of the operator and the difficulty of the procedure.

In most circumstances, time is allowed between extraction of teeth and placement of the fixture. In patients with moderately or advanced periodontal disease where the degree of bone loss is significant, extraction of teeth may result in more bone loss. Placement of the fixture at the time of extraction can preserve the bone and maintain the gingival architecture. However, the position of the fixture by necessity must be in the same location as the tooth and therefore there is little flexibility in re-positioning the fixture.

● Bridge abutments

Bridge abutments will differ slightly from the single-tooth abutment because the need to prevent anti-rotational forces is not as great. Linking the bridge between abutments will effectively prevent rotational forces being significant. However, the operator must choose the optimum number of implants to span the edentulous space. This does not mean that each tooth need be replaced by an implant. Two implants linked to a three-unit bridge can replace three missing teeth. Larger spans may increase the risk for failure. There is a myriad of abutments available, depending upon the fixture manufacturer, the position of the bridge and the appearance and depth of the fixture head.

● Overdenture abutments

Traditionally, a bar, ball or magnet has been used to link the denture to the abutment (see Fig. 14.3). The abutments are placed so that they are surrounded by the greatest amount of bone; this usually means in the canine or premolar region. This also allows the optimum support for a denture, being mid-way between the posterior and anterior edentulous jaw. As common with any overdenture, the interocclusal space is fundamental because thin dentures will fracture under load, especially when opposed by teeth or implants.

Ball fixtures fit into a female part within the denture, which are made with either a metal or plastic ring. Magnets, which are preferred by some operators, have good early retention, but the strength of the magnet can decay over time and reduce the retention. Some dentists prefer bars, especially in the anterior mandible, which are inserted into metal tags attached to the fit surface of the denture.

Learning outcomes

- Understanding bone grafts for implants.
- Choosing the optimum number of implants.
- Implant impression techniques.
- Types of abutments.
- Typical characteristics of implant systems.

Further reading

Davenport J, Basker R, Heath J et al 2000 A clinical guide to removable partial dentures. BDJ Books, London

Grant A, Johnson W 1992 Removable prosthodontics. Churchill Livingstone, Edinburgh

Ibbetson R, Eder A 2000 Tooth surface loss. BDJ Books, London

McCabe J, Walls A 1998 Applied dental materials, 8th edn. Blackwell Science, Edinburgh

Palmer R, Smith B, Howe L, Palmer P 2002 Implants in clinical dentistry. Martin Dunitz, London

Smith BGN 1998 Planning and making crowns and bridges, 3rd edn. Martin Dunitz, London

Smith B, Wright P, Brown D 1994 The clinical handling of dental materials, 2nd edn. Butterworth Heinemann, Oxford

Walmsley A, Walsh T, Burke T et al 2002 Restorative dentistry. Churchill Livingstone, Edinburgh

Wassell R, Walls A, Steele J et al 2002 A clinical guide to crowns and other extra-coronal restorations. BDJ Books, London

Index

Page numbers in *italics* refer to figures and boxes.